The Politics of COVID-19 in Mexico

This book evaluates the factors behind Mexico's painful experience with the COVID-19 crisis, a country that ranked fifth in the world for the number of deaths caused by the virus. Through a series of vignettes, its authors point to pandemic politics as the culprit. With a focus on the nexus of global governance and government in the Mexican case, they underline the politicised nature of domestic, international, and transnational responses to the pandemic. The chapters analyse the multiple political dimensions that affected the ability of intergovernmental and governmental authorities to construct timely, effective, and equitable health security against the COVID-19 virus, including symbolic politics, medical populism, global political economy, disease diplomacy, epistemic communities, and federalism. This volume builds an interdisciplinary analysis of the politics of pandemic governance, bridging political science, international relations, public policy and public administration, and public health.

Thomas Legler is a research professor of International Relations at the Universidad Iberoamericana in Mexico City, and a member of the National System of Researchers in Mexico, level III. His research focuses on regional governance and institutions in Latin America. He holds a Ph.D. in Political Science from York University (Toronto).

The Politics of COVID-19 in Mexico: Governance
Meets Government

https://www.routledge.com/The-Politics-of-Pandemics/book-series/TPOP

The Politics of COVID-19 in Mexico

Governance Meets Government

Thomas Legler

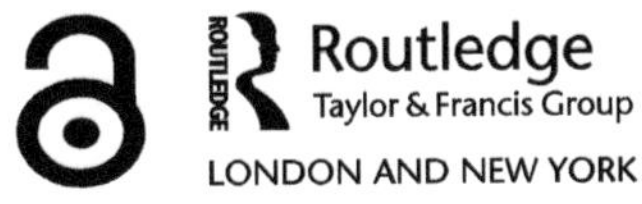

Routledge
Taylor & Francis Group

LONDON AND NEW YORK

First published 2025
by Routledge
4 Park Square, Milton Park, Abingdon, Oxon OX14 4RN

and by Routledge
605 Third Avenue, New York, NY 10158

Routledge is an imprint of the Taylor & Francis Group, an informa business

British Library Cataloguing-in-Publication Data
A catalogue record for this book is available from the British Library

ISBN: 978-1-032-73797-3 (hbk)
ISBN: 978-1-032-80002-8 (pbk)
ISBN: 978-1-003-49495-9 (ebk)

DOI: 10.4324/9781003494959

Typeset in Sabon
by Apex CoVantage, LLC

Contents

Figures

Tables

Contributors

Caroline Irene Deschak
Senior Nutrition and Food Security
    Research Specialist, ICF
Rockville, MD, USA

Laura Zamudio González
Professor of International Relations,
    Department of International Relations
    Universidad Iberoamericana
Mexico Cit, Mexico

Thomas Legler
Professor of International Relations,
    Department of International Stud-
    ies Universidad Iberoamericana
Mexico City, Mexico

Ricardo Velázquez Leyer
Professor of Public Policy, Depart-
    ment of Social and Political Sci-
    ences Universidad Iberoamericana
Mexico City, Mexico

María Esther Coronado Martínez
Lecturer, School of Law National
    Autonomous University of Mexico
    (UNAM)
Mexico City, Mexico

María Gabriela Palacio Ludeña
Assistant Professor in Development
    Studies, Latin American Studies
    Programme Leiden University
Leiden, Netherlands

Heidi Jane M. Smith
Professor of Economics, Department
    of Economics
Universidad Iberoamericana
Mexico City, Mexico

Michelle Ruiz Valdes
Sessional Lecturer, Department of
    International Studies Universidad
    Iberoamericana
Mexico City, Mexico

Valeria Marina Valle
Professor of International Relations,
    Department of International Stud-
    ies and the Center for Critical
    Gender and Feminism Studies
    (CECRIGE) Universidad Ibero-
    americana
Mexico City, Mexico

Preface

The idea for this book was conceived in the early months of the COVID-19 pandemic, when my wife and I found ourselves confined to our apartment on the fifteenth floor of a residential building in the Miraflores district of Lima. What had started as a dream sabbatical for us at the Pontifical Catholic University of Peru in the first week of March 2020 became a months-long ordeal of restricted mobility in the context of Peru's strict national lockdown. As a monumental, emotional, and watershed occurrence with such a personalised impact in my own life, I felt drawn and compelled as a scholar of International Relations with a keen interest in global governance to try to make sense of the problematic collective responses to the pandemic during those months of confinement in Peru.

As luck would have it, I soon found funding to pursue my newfound interest in the global governance of the COVID-19 pandemic. During spring 2020, my university, the Universidad Iberoamericana, launched an in-house call for proposals for interdisciplinary research projects on the COVID-19 crisis. I quickly put together a team of friends and colleagues from across three different departments and disciplines at the Ibero who shared my passion and concern for this game changer in our lives: Heidi Smith (Department of Economics), Valeria Valle (Department of International Studies), Ricardo Velázquez (Department of Social and Political Sciences), and Laura Zamudio (Department of International Studies). Together, we submitted a successful funding proposal entitled "The Global Governance of Health Security in Mexico in the Context of the COVID-19 Pandemic." As the research project that became this book evolved, it grew to include additional collaborators and co-authors: María Esther Coronado (Faculty of Law, National Autonomous University of Mexico), Caroline Deschak (EQUIDE, Universidad Iberoamericana), María Gabriela Palacio (Latin American Studies Programme, Universiteit Leiden), and Michelle Ruiz (Department of International Studies, Universidad Iberoamericana).

Mexico occupied fifth place in the world in terms of the number of people killed by the disease. It was also the country with the highest number of deaths among doctors and health workers, and among the worst for orphaned children. At the core of this collective effort is our shared interest in explaining this painful experience. As we stress in these pages, this fiasco was avoidable. In our search for explanations, we wanted to move beyond simplistic and methodologically nationalistic arguments that solely put the blame on the role of Mexican authorities. Our focus was on the nexus of global governance and government in the response to the pandemic in Mexican territory, hence the title of the book. Our respective chapters underscore that the weak performance against COVID-19 in Mexico was in large part because global governors and domestic authorities all too often got the politics of pandemics wrong. The authors in this volume detail how a variety of diverse forms of pandemic politics detracted from efforts to construct health security in the midst of the crisis, including disease diplomacy; the relationship between the Mexican government and the World Health Organization; the global political economy of pandemic governance; the politics of epistemic communities; vaccine populism; and the politics of federalism.

This book would not have been possible without the help of numerous individuals. First, the authors would like to thank the Universidad Iberoamericana for its generous financial support. Marisol Silva, Jimena de Gortari, and the rest of the team at the Research and Graduate Directorate (DINVP) were instrumental in awarding us a generous grant through the #IBEROFRENTEALCOVID19 competition, as well as through their continuous administrative support. Alejandro Anaya, Graciela Teruel, and Luis González saw to it that we received additional backing to offer this volume as open access. Graciela Ramírez was the administrative lynchpin for the day-to-day budgetary transactions for our project.

A small army of research assistants helped me research and write my chapter as well as bring this book to life. In this regard, I would like to recognise the contributions of Jessy Quezada, Paula Mariana González, Ximena Villafaña, Paulina Robles, Mariana Romo, Mariana Kiimi Ortiz, and Rubén Mendoza. Others, both authors in this volume and colleagues and friends, made important contributions to the book through the feedback that they provided on select chapters: Laura Zamudio, David Arellano, María Esther Coronado, and Ricardo Velázquez.

Special thanks go to the team at Routledge for all their support and guidance, from the original book proposal through the process that brought this book to fruition. Rob Sorsby was key in this regard. We are grateful to the external reviewers selected by Routledge, Jorge Schiavon, and Élodie Brun for their green light and helpful comments. The usual disclaimer applies: Any shortcomings in this volume are ours and not theirs. Thank you to Raj Nandini, Ananya Girdhar, and Aruna Rajendran for their assistance with the contractual, copy editing, and production process.

Behind the scenes, my wife, Noemi Vidal, deserves a lot of credit for her unwavering support during the lengthy ordeal that produced this publication. She stood by me through the long weeks and months that went into this project; I could not have done this without her.

On a final note, we, the authors, sincerely hope that this volume makes a modest contribution to the critical yet constructive literature whose goal is to learn from the mistakes of the collective responses to the COVID-19 pandemic so as not to repeat them in the future, for no doubt there will be future deadly outbreaks. In the memory of all those who did not survive the scourge of COVID-19, this book is dedicated to helping get the pandemic politics right the next time around.

Thomas Legler

1 Introduction

Governance Meets Government: The Pandemic Politics of Mexico's Response to the COVID-19 Virus

Thomas Legler

Mexico's Painful Experience With COVID-19: The Search for Answers

At the outset of the COVID-19 pandemic in early 2020, Mexico found itself in a similar predicament to many other countries across the planet. Its public health system was ill-prepared for what was to come (see GHS Index, 2019; Global Preparedness Monitoring Board, 2019). Against an unknown corona-virus whose global reach and magnitude were unprecedented, it confronted the daunting and urgent challenge of how to fill a series of governance gaps—informational, policy, normative, institutional, and compliance—in order to control the virus, protect its population, and manage the multiple health and non-health-related dimensions of the crisis.[1] To make matters even worse, in their efforts to construct and bolster health security against the virus in record time,[2] import-dependent countries like Mexico, with more limited human, scientific, medical, technological, and economic resource endow-ments, found themselves hard hit by global supply shocks brought on by a wave of national lockdowns and travel restrictions.

On May 5, 2023, roughly three and a half years after the COVID-19 virus first spread across the planet, Dr. Tedros Adhanom Ghebreyesus, Direc-tor General of the World Health Organization (WHO), announced that the COVID-19 pandemic no longer constituted a public health emergency of international concern (PHEIC). Despite the similar situation and challenges that so many countries faced at its beginning, with the benefit of hindsight, we can now see that Mexico's experience managing this global health crisis was particularly painful. In absolute terms, in May 2023, Mexico's official death count due to the virus, approximately 334,000, was the fifth highest in the world (see Figure 1.1).

Mexico's mortality rate is even more alarming when the number of excess deaths is taken into account. In this regard, diverse sources indicate that during 2020–2021, COVID-19 was the leading cause of death and that Mexico was among the top seven countries in terms of excess mortality rate (Miranda, 2022; Palacio-Mejía *et al.*, 2022; Wang *et al.*, 2022). According

DOI: 10.4324/9781003494959-1

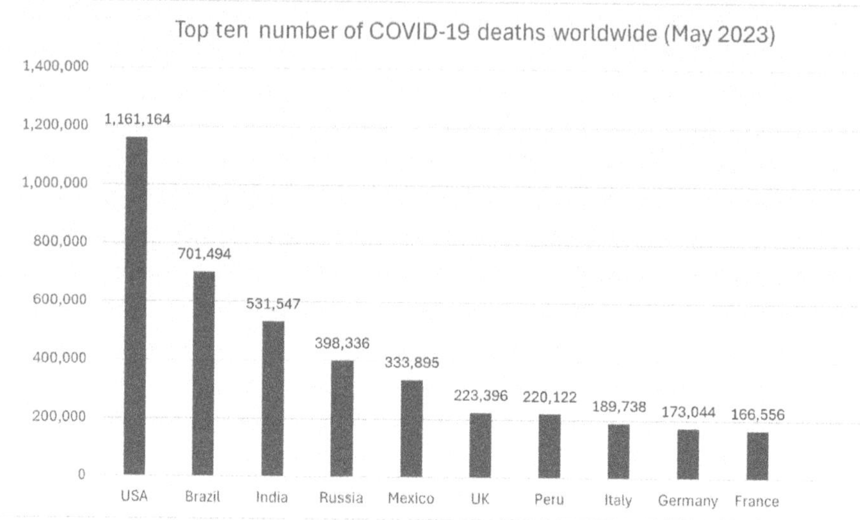

Figure 1.1 Top ten number of COVID-19 deaths worldwide (May 2023)

Source: Statista Search Department (May 2, 2023) *Number of novel coronavirus (COVID-19) deaths worldwide as of May 2, 2023, by country and territory* [Chart]. Statista. www.statista.com/statistics/1093256/novel-coronavirus-2019ncov-deaths-worldwide-by-country/

to one estimate, Mexico suffered 202,141 COVID-19-related excess deaths in 2020 and a further 237,441 in 2021 (Palacio-Mejía *et al.*, 2022, p. 4). With 4,084 deaths by early 2022, the country also established an international record early on in the pandemic for the highest number of public and private health workers who succumbed to the illness (Hernández-Ruiz *et al.*, 2022). Moreover, more than 215,000 children were orphaned because of COVID-19, among the eight most affected states on the planet (Sánchez Talanquer and Sepúlveda, 2024, p. 82). In the first two years of the pandemic, hospitals were repeatedly overwhelmed by the public demand created by the high rate of infection, barring many seriously ill patients from hospitalisation or causing them to die waiting for hospital beds to free up on nearby sidewalks or parking lots, or in their beds at home. In retrospect, many Mexican deaths were undeniably preventable.

How do we explain that despite a similar starting point at the beginning of the pandemic in relation to other countries, Mexico would turn out to have among the most problematic records in terms of human costs and suffering? Undoubtedly, there is no single or simple answer to this question. A number of critical analyses assign blame to domestic variables linked to the problematic handling of the pandemic by the Mexican government (Lizárraga and Suárez, 2022; De la Cerda and Martínez-Gallardo, 2023; Moreno, 2022; Sánchez Talanquer and Sepúlveda, 2024; Sánchez Talanquer *et al.*, 2021; Velázquez Leyer, 2021; Ximénez-Fyvie, 2021, 2022). These critiques identify and underline a litany of questionable policy choices and measures that often contradicted or disregarded the public health recommendations of the WHO: Ignoring valuable experience gained from Mexico's experience with the H1N1 epidemic in 2009; the implementation of a sentinel surveillance system at the expense of mass testing; the absence of process-tracing; a minimalist overall response; the slow adoption of masks and social distancing; advocating personal responsibility and voluntary public compliance with mitigation measures rather than strict enforcement; the marginalisation of the General Health Council and the National Health Council in favour of centralised health crisis management; a questionable epidemiological traffic light system; lax quarantine measures; weak screening of incoming international travellers; and limited public expenditure to combat the virus.

In a similar vein, the analysis of Jennifer Cyr and her collaborators makes a direct link in countries like Mexico between the relative lack of "collaborative governance" and alarming death rates due to COVID-19 (Cyr *et al.*, 2021). In other words, Latin American governments that did not exercise significant cooperation and coordination with diverse public, private, and non-governmental actors across different jurisdictional levels in their pandemic responses generally fared far worse in terms of deaths caused. A common thread through various chapters in this book is that Mexican authorities failed to mobilise a whole-of-government and whole-of-society approach to combatting the virus and its multiple repercussions (see Chapters 3 and 5).

Rather than managing the multidimensional COVID-19 crisis effectively, Mexico's public policy responses exacerbated a series of vulnerabilities that existed prior to the outbreak. These included a fragmented, underfunded, underequipped, and undersupplied national public health system; pronounced social inequalities; and widespread comorbidities such as diabetes, obesity, and heart disease that rendered the pandemic simultaneously a syndemic (Gamlin *et al.*, 2021; Lustig and Mariscal, 2021; Sánchez Talanquer *et al.*, 2021; Sánchez Talanquer and Sepúlveda, 2024; Singer, 2020; Singer *et al.*, 2017).

Although the authors whose chapters appear in this volume draw on this important literature and subscribe to its criticisms, they present collectively a different approach that not only includes but also goes beyond the national policy and administrative framework in terms of seeking to account for the problematic health security performance in Mexico against the COVID-19 pandemic. As the title of this book suggests, *Governance Meets Government*, although Mexican authorities share the blame for the aforementioned debacle, their actions did not occur in a vacuum. They happened in interaction with a host of other actors and organisations in the Western Hemisphere and at the global level, and within the framework of a regional and global health governance architecture. Recent official reports underscore the shortcomings of the responses of the WHO and other authoritative intergovernmental, transnational, and private actors and how they impacted negatively on national efforts across the planet to combat COVID-19 (see Global

Preparedness Monitoring Board, 2020, 2021; Independent Panel, 2021; Sirleaf and Clark, 2022). In other words, international and transnational causal factors are also potentially significant in terms of explaining what transpired in Mexico during the pandemic. Accordingly, the analyses herein seek to understand how *the nexus* of specific and tangible (global) governance and governmental actors, institutions, and processes affected the experience of the pandemic on Mexican soil.[3]

The analysis of Mexico's trials with COVID-19 as a governance meets government problematic is reinforced by the pandemic's nature as a wicked problem.[4] That is, from both a public policy and a broader global governance perspective, the pandemic is a public problem that is exceedingly difficult to solve, let alone manage, due to its social, epidemiological, political, economic, temporal, and spatial complexity. Indeed, according to some scholars, like climate change, it merits the designation of *super wicked problem* (Auld *et al.*, 2021). From the angle of its (super) wickedness, a methodologically nationalist framework that focuses on explaining Mexico's experience *vis-à-vis* the global COVID-19 crisis as a public policy and administration problematic is simply inadequate on its own.

In attempting to comprehend Mexico's dismal COVID-19 record, the other tie that binds the authors in this volume is the important role that they attribute to *pandemic politics*. As has been made abundantly clear by international social and news media, global and regional governance, coupled with the domestic public management of the COVID-19 crisis, have been intensely political processes (see also Boin *et al.*, 2021).

The COVID-19 experience has spawned an impressive and growing number of book-length studies under the rubric of pandemic politics, each with a different emphasis. Indeed, this volume forms part of a new series under Routledge by the same name. In terms of the eclecticism that characterises this research, according to Aaltola (2012, 2022), pandemics are highly disruptive "politosomatic" phenomena that unleash fear and anxiety throughout interconnected individual, bodily, and political levels and across globalised geographies. In *Viral Lobbying*, Crepaz *et al.* (2022) focus on the politics of interest groups and lobbying during the COVID-19 crisis. Bringel and Pleyers (2022) target the global politics of states, social movements, and civil society in the face of the virus. Kushner Gadarian, Wallace Goodman, and Pepinsky (2022) equate pandemic politics with the polarised, partisan politics that plagued the US response to COVID-19 in 2020. Kahl and Wright (2021) underline how COVID-19 became a truly global political crisis with far-reaching circumstances that included a coup de grace for the existing international order. Undoubtedly, all of these disparate analytical strands enrich our understanding and appreciation of the multiple political dimensions of pandemics like that of COVID-19.

Following Nunes' (2014) exploration of the politics of health security, a holistic and comprehensive treatment of pandemic politics would ideally comprise three components: its political nature; its political impact; and its political potential. However, when we refer to governance meets government, our emphasis is in particular on specific *procedural* and *instrumental* aspects of the politics of pandemic responses. How do political processes shape those responses, and how do they affect governance or governmental performance? The chapters herein underscore that pandemic politics entails a multiplicity of politicised interactions that occur at and across multiple spatial levels among the diverse actors whose actions or inaction shape responses to contagious disease outbreaks. The authors in this text suggest that in numerous instances, governance and governmental actors, both Mexican and non-Mexican, within the Mexican context got the politics of governance and government wrong, with often tragic human consequences. In what follows, I flesh out a set of common patterns that underpin our own analyses of the politics of pandemics, as experienced on Mexican soil.

Pandemic Politics: International Patterns and Mexican Vignettes

As is to be expected, the political dimensions of Mexico's experience managing the COVID-19 crisis reflect both common international trends and *sui generis*, made in Mexico elements. In what follows, this section is divided into two parts. First, it looks at common patterns of pandemic politics identified in the literature on global health governance, both prior to and during COVID-19, and some of their recent manifestations in Mexico. Second, it presents a summary of the contributions of each chapter to our understanding of the pandemic politics of COVID-19 in Mexico. Each author or set of co-authors focuses their analysis on a specific case, providing us with a series of detailed vignettes that illuminate crucial political components of the struggle against the virus as it was experienced in this country. The chapters highlight the multiplicity, texture, and nuance of the political factors that have influenced the management of the COVID-19 crisis in Mexico's case, undoubtedly valuable for the study of pandemic politics in other contexts.

International Patterns of Pandemic Politics

Well before the global COVID-19 outbreak, a number of studies based on prior PHEICs had already recognised that pandemic responses were rife with politics (see, e.g. Bjørkdahl and Carlsen, 2019; Davies and Youde, 2015). As de Bengy Puyvallée and Kittelsen (2018) stressed, pandemic preparedness and response are both technical and political matters. On the basis of their evaluation of the H1N1 virus, Ebola, and Zika public health emergencies, Hoffmann and Silverberg (2018) noted that both technical surveillance problems and political factors caused important time delays in necessary collective action to confront these viruses.

The course of events during the COVID-19 pandemic has borne out the cruciality of getting politics right and the risk of getting them wrong. As Thomas Hale and his collaborators (Hale *et al.*, 2021, p. 2) have noted,

> Throughout the COVID-19 crisis, political dynamics have been amongst the most powerful drivers of health outcomes globally, nationally, and locally. Geopolitical tensions have made it more difficult to coordinate across countries, and domestic tensions have reduced the effectiveness of national responses.

Jennie Gamlin and her co-authors (2021, p. 4) are even more blunt: "[P]olitics is a primary structural determinant of COVID-19 mortality." In light of recent events, Cousins *et al.* (2021) assert that global health is a political enterprise.

A quick glance at the vast literature on the subject suggests at least five areas where pandemic politics that involve interactions between global governance and governments can negatively affect health crisis outcomes: symbolic politics; disease diplomacy; the politics of compliance with the 2005 International Health Regulations (IHR); medical populism; and the international political economy of contagious diseases.

First, pandemic responses entail symbolic politics. According to Louise Comfort and her co-authors (Comfort, 2007, 2022; Comfort *et al.*, 2020), the ability to mount collective action against any crisis requires the construction of collective cognition, or the shared recognition of a threat, and the ability to create that shared meaning through effective communication among diverse actors. This process is highly politicised. In the tradition of Foucault, diseases and pandemics are political experiences that are constructed symbolically through political communications and accordingly can take on diverse connotations with different political ends (Nunes, 2014). From a crisis management perspective, governments attempt to frame the pandemic in ways that make sense of the threat and create credible narratives, but in the context of highly politicised framing contests with other actors (Boin, McConnell and Hart, 2021). Leach and Tadros (2014) assert that diverse actors typically construct multiple, competing narratives during epidemics.

In the first few months of the coronavirus outbreak, the efforts of the WHO to construct collective cognition as the basis for coordinated collective action were severely hampered by symbolic politics. While the WHO sought to alert the global public to the emergency and dangers of COVID-19 and to galvanise action accordingly, many national authorities offered a completely different, less severe, and less urgent risk assessment. During the early months of the outbreak, it was common across a number of countries, including Mexico, for public health authorities, politicians, and presidents to downplay the risks and severity of the virus (on Mexico, see Lizárraga and Suárez, 2022; Sánchez Talanquer *et al.*, 2021; Sánchez Talanquer and Sepúlveda, 2024; Velázquez Leyer, 2021; Ximénez-Fyvie, 2021). Similarly, some critics assert that President López Obrador devised a policy narrative during the COVID-19 crisis that intentionally downplayed or limited scientific expertise and advanced his own personal political agenda and personal biases at the expense of providing an adequate explanation and appropriate policies (Peci, Dussauge-Laguna and González, 2022).

By a similar token, symbolic politics hurt efforts by public health authorities at the WHO and across many countries to promote vaccination against COVID-19. They were frequently hampered by what became known as an *infodemic*: "too much information including false or misleading information in digital and physical environments during a disease outbreak" (World Health Organization, n.d.; see also Zarocostas, 2020). The often confusing and contradictory information provided to the public via diverse media contributed to a phenomenon that the WHO labelled vaccine hesitancy. This problem underscored the enormous, politically sensitive challenge confronting health professionals in terms of crafting effective *messaging* in contexts where public trust was vulnerable to misinformation and political manipulation (on the importance of messaging, see Council of the Americas, 2023). Although Mexico's own experience with vaccine hesitancy was not as profound as in many other countries, the spread of false information through social media caused a number of unfortunate incidents during the initial months of the pandemic, in which medical personnel were physically attacked on various occasions for their perceived role in propagating the virus, as were other health workers for spraying disinfectants across different municipalities (see González Díaz, 2020).

A second arena of pandemic politics is "disease diplomacy": diplomatic efforts and interactions involving a host of state, intergovernmental, and non-state actors in the global system of disease surveillance and control (Davies, Kamradt-Scott and Rushton, 2015). With a focus on different types of negotiations and other interactions involved in international public health issues, the three-part taxonomy developed by Rebecca Katz and her collaborators (2011) for the broader notion of global health diplomacy gives a good idea of the universe of possibilities for disease diplomacy and the actors involved: core or formal diplomacy (high politics); multistakeholder diplomacy; and informal diplomacy (Katz *et al.*, 2011; see also Ruckert *et al.*, 2016).

Certainly, Mexican actors were quite active in disease diplomacy during the pandemic. For instance, in terms of high politics, Mexican foreign ministry officials, including the ambassador to the United Nations (U.N.), Juan Ramón de la Fuente, were instrumental in coordinating a coalition of 120 countries that advocated for the equitable access of countries of the Global South to medicines, medical equipment, and vaccines. Mexico's efforts culminated in UN General Assembly Resolution 74/274 (Legler, 2021). Multistakeholder and informal diplomacy were evident in both the complex negotiations and interactions that led to a public-private partnership among Mexican and Argentinian governmental, non-governmental, and private actors, the multinational pharmaceutical company AstraZeneca, and Oxford University to produce and distribute COVID-19 vaccines.

However, the politics of disease diplomacy also took some less fortunate and twisted directions during the COVID-19 pandemic. In the context of worldwide supply shortages and heightened geopolitical rivalry among China, the European Union, Russia, and the United States, these countries first engaged at the onset of the outbreak in mask diplomacy, the bilateral donation of protective masks to poorer countries for soft power ends, followed subsequently by vaccine diplomacy (with a similar logic). In the latter case, the politicised practice by vaccine-producing countries of giving gifts of vaccines to countries of the Global South rather than to the newly established COVAX facility undermined this global vaccine mechanism's efforts to establish itself as an effective and exclusive global buyers' pool that could offer affordable and equitable access to vaccines across the planet (see Chapter 3 in this volume).

A third area of pandemic politics is the politics of compliance with and implementation of the 2005 International Health Regulations (IHR) in public health emergency situations (see, e.g. Davies and Youde, 2015). As Jonathan E. Suk (2007, p. 2) has noted, "During a pandemic, science and politics are difficult to disentangle." As he observed with respect to the 2003 SARS pandemic, novel PHEIC, especially at their outset, can be moments marked by the absence of reliable and proven scientific knowledge to anchor WHO's recommendations for mitigation measures. These moments of uncertainty can be potentially exploited by diverse actors for political ends. Concerned about the economic consequences and political fallout of following WHO's recommendations, governments may use the lack of scientific certainty to resist their obligations under the IHR in favour of measures that are more politically palatable for their populations. In other words, WHO's epidemic responses under the IHR are vulnerable to politicisation.

As various chapters echo in this book, this was certainly evident in Mexico's experience with COVID-19. As already suggested earlier, in an initial context of serious scientific knowledge and information gaps, Mexican authorities complied with WHO's recommendations on a select or delayed basis throughout much of the pandemic. For example, the Mexican government was slow to advocate the use of masks and social distancing. It also failed to adopt significant testing or process tracing regimes.

Fourth, in an almost prophetic way, Lasco and Curato (2019) wrote just months before the COVID-19 pandemic that health crises are susceptible to politicisation and in particular to a political phenomenon that they termed medical populism. Following their definition, medical populism is "a political style that constructs antagonistic relations between 'the people' whose lives have been put at risk by 'the establishment'" (Lasco and Curato, 2019, p. 1). According to their analysis, medical populism is characterised by an appeal by the leader to the people pitted against a medical or scientific establishment and the construction of a health crisis as a dramatised performance based on a simplified discourse.

The number of empirical cases of medical populism during the COVID-19 pandemic abounded, including US President Donald Trump, Philippine President Rodrigo Duterte, and Brazilian President Jair Bolsonaro (see Lancet COVID-19 Commission, 2020; Lasco, 2020; Ringe and Rennó, 2023; Roberts, 2022). The actions of these leaders often frustrated the attempts by public health authorities, health workers, researchers, and medical specialists to develop effective science-based measures and, on a number of occasions, had devastating consequences in terms of human infection, illness, and death. For example, through their actions and personal, symbolic conduct, these practitioners of medical populism impeded the rapid and widespread adoption of simple, cheap, and effective mitigation measures such as the use of masks and social distancing (Lancet COVID-19 Commission, 2020). Indeed, various studies have posited that populist governments performed significantly worse in protecting their populations against COVID-19 than those who deferred to public health and medical specialists and scientific evidence in the design and implementation of their responses (Bayerlein *et al.*, 2021; Hanson and Kopstein, 2021; Sánchez Talanquer and Sepúlveda, 2024, p. 29; Touchton *et al.*, 2023).

President López Obrador of Mexico has been severely criticised for his role in promoting medical populism during the pandemic (De la Cerda and Martínez-Gallardo, 2023; Gómez Dantés and Frenk Mora, 2020; Rentería and Arellano-Gault, 2021). He downplayed the seriousness of the epidemic in the initial months of the pandemic, claiming before the media that COVID-19 was less harmful than influenza. While public health authorities across the country sought to promote public adherence to mitigation measures, for many months López Obrador appeared in public without wearing a mask and attended mass public rallies with little or no social distancing and in close contact with his multitude of followers.

Yet as De la Cerda and Martínez-Gallardo (2023) have observed, despite these antics, the overall slowness, laxity and underfunding of Mexican governmental measures, and the severity of the impact of the virus on the Mexican population, the response was politically very effective. López Obrador maintained relatively high rates of popular approval, and his political party, MORENA, retained a simple majority in the 2021 congressional midterm elections and won 11 out of 15 gubernatorial contests. López Obrador's variant of medical populism promoted a selective adoption of recommendations from the WHO and scientific experts, a centralisation of pandemic decision-making at the expense of a more horizontal, consultative, and coordinated approach through the General Health Council and the National Health Council, and the persistent promotion of social and political polarisation instead of national unity.

Finally, a fifth way to conceptualise pandemic politics is as an international political economy problematic. For many years, critics have pointed out how the juxtaposition of capitalism and public health has produced gross health inequities across the planet, from the local to the global level. Farmer's (1999, 2003) pathbreaking work underlined how domestic and global disparities in political and economic power have sustained structural violence in both developed and underdeveloped countries that includes serious inequalities in access to public health and medical care, as well as systematic violations of the social and economic rights of the poor and marginalised. These "pathologies of power and powerlessness" (Farmer, 1999, 2003) in turn have had pathogenic effects in terms of the human suffering caused by communicable and non-communicable diseases on societies' most vulnerable populations. In recent years, two important international commissions concluded that the dysfunctions of global governance for health share much of the blame for this unacceptable and unequal status quo (Ottersen *et al.*, 2014; World Health Organization, 2008). Global health governance has played an important role in the maldistribution of economic, medical, productive, intellectual, normative, and political resources required to promote more equitable access to public health both within countries and across the divide between the Global North and the Global South.

Not surprisingly, the COVID-19 pandemic exposed and exacerbated this state of affairs (Gamlin *et al.*, 2021; Hennis *et al.*, 2021; Lancet COVID-19 Commission, 2020). As historically has been the case, this pandemic hit the so-called *precariat* the hardest, that is, the structurally most vulnerable living on the fringes of society (Daher-Nashif, 2021; Gamlin *et al.*, 2021; Hennis *et al.*, 2021). Global responses to the virus also reinforced the North-South divide (Cousins *et al.*, 2021; Gamlin *et al.*, 2021). Despite rhetoric about the need to promote global public goods to strengthen health security everywhere, the countries of the Global North frequently used their political and economic clout to procure their own supplies of medical equipment, supplies, medicines, and vaccines at the expense of WHO's efforts and the Global South. The development and commercialisation of medicines and vaccines to combat the virus also once again disproportionately benefitted multinational pharmaceutical companies of the Global North.

The global political economy of the pandemic was more than evident in Mexico's experience. Although officially the targeted beneficiaries of AMLO's Fourth Transformation, pandemic politics undoubtedly exacerbated the vulnerability of Mexico's poor to COVID-19. Socioeconomic inequality fostered differential access to hospitalisation, medication, vaccines, and COVID-19 testing, and the greater prevalence of comorbidities such as obesity, diabetes, and heart disease made those in poverty more vulnerable to serious illness and death. On the international front, as Chapter 3 underlines, despite paying in advance for vaccines through the WHO's new COVAX facility, the Mexican government found itself struggling with more politically and economically powerful Western countries to obtain an adequate supply for its population.

The Pandemic Politics of COVID-19: Mexican Vignettes

As mentioned beforehand, the six chapters that follow in this book offer critical explorations of the pandemic politics associated with the juxtaposition of global governance and government in the struggle against COVID-19 in Mexican territorial space. The vignettes they offer illustrate the patterns identified in the previous section as well as present additional aspects of pandemic politics that influence governance outcomes. In general, the chapters have been ordered according to their respective level of governance, from the global to the local.

In Chapter 2, Laura Zamudio's contribution investigates the challenges and problems involved in integrating a coordinated response between the WHO and the Mexican government during the pandemic. She examines the highly politicised process of filling in multiple governance gaps through cooperation, or the lack thereof, between the two. According to Zamudio, Mexico's experience was marked by a profound disagreement or rift and minimal coordination between the WHO and the López Obrador government—a political divergence that actually culminated in the creation of new governance gaps rather than the filling in of existing ones. Symbolic politics and medical populism seriously impeded a more propitious relationship between the two and, importantly, revealed the limits of orchestration by international organisations *vis-à-vis* populist governments. Moreover, the select disagreement and minimal coordination between the two prevented a shared understanding of the nature and severity of the phenomenon. She calls for more attention to the development of organisational strategies by international organisations that diminish political discord in managing global crises and support the execution of essential functions such as providing meaning (a shared understanding of the nature of the threat) and control (strategies for action, methods, and rationales).

In Chapter 3, Esther Coronado adds another significant analytical dimension to pandemic politics: the politicisation and politics of epistemic communities during the pandemic. Mexico's experience underlines that these transnational networks are often politicised through the dual role that scientists often play as experts and bureaucrats. Although epistemic communities are supposed to work as dissemination mechanisms for crucial technical and scientific ideas during international health crises, she explores why they have often failed to disseminate global policy recommendations to manage the COVID-19 pandemic. Crucial in her analysis is how, through the overlap of epistemic communities and transgovernmental networks, and as personified in the figure of Hugo López-Gatell Ramírez, Mexico's undersecretary of health and COVID-19 tsar, global governance via the WHO became enmeshed with domestic politics. Crucially, through their vulnerability to politicisation, expert groups can use their role as authorities on an issue to promote a political ideology even if it does not resonate with science. In light of Mexico's travails, she contends that epistemic communities have had to vie with the increased politicisation of some of their key members, causing weaknesses and fractures in their networks' internal structures, thus affecting their ability to promote global policy transfer.

In Chapter 4, Thomas Legler analyses Mexico's experience with the politics of vaccination against the COVID-19 virus. His contribution seeks to explain the country's lacklustre record with respect to the immunisation of its population, as captured in comparative statistics, significant delays in the crucial first year of the vaccine roll-out in 2021, the initial exclusion of important population segments like private sector doctors and health workers, people with comorbidities, and children, as well as the acquisition and application of vaccines of dubious reliability. He finds that the shortcomings in this regard can be attributed to the juxtaposition of the prevailing global political economy of vaccine governance and the Mexican government's adoption of a populist vaccine strategy. That is, COVID-19 revealed that despite rhetoric to the contrary, the emerging global pandemic vaccine governance complex favoured the interests of countries and pharmaceutical companies of the Global North, fostering vaccine inequity rather than more equitable access to vaccines. Confronted with how to obtain a timely, adequate, and effective supply of vaccines and to apply them urgently, Mexican authorities responded in a highly centralised and politicised manner that sacrificed a more comprehensive whole-of-government and whole-of-society approach.

Valeria Marina Valle, Caroline Irene Deschak, and Michelle Ruíz Valdes analyse the multilevel governance (MLG) of health security with a focus on migrant access to health services in one key border region between Mexico and the United States: Tijuana and San Diego. Their analysis highlights two important dimensions of pandemic politics at the local level. On the one hand, they delve into the limits of formal disease diplomacy by governmental actors for the construction of migrant access to health services on the border during the pandemic and the importance of informal networks of disease diplomacy involving public, non-governmental, and private actors. On the other hand, their research also utilises elements of critical and feminist political economy, confirming that COVID-19 is above all a pandemic of inequalities. In this regard, migrants are not only one of the most disadvantaged groups but also one that is a heterogeneous category along intersectional lines whose members have experienced differential institutional discrimination and access to health services. Migrant vulnerability is far from homogeneous; greater risks were detected when taking into account age, gender, and other identities. Their chapter underscores the complexity of health responses in border contexts during the pandemic and highlights the urgent need for a more effective multilevel governance approach and integrative disease diplomacy to address health inequalities and advance towards the achievement of Sustainable Development Goals 3, 10, and 17.

In their analysis, María Gabriela Palacio Ludeña and Ricardo Velázquez Leyer compare the problematic linkage between global policy and the resilience of national health systems in Mexico and Ecuador. Drawing on diverse forms of pandemic politics, they underscore the political limits of responses on both sides of the equation: intergovernmental organisations and governments. Ideally, global policy ought to steer national decision-making processes since the adoption of emergency measures devised with the knowledge generated by intergovernmental and transnational actors is fundamental to protecting people's well-being. However, their comparison reveals the contradictions and limitations of global policy diffusion during the COVID-19 pandemic. On the one hand, Ecuador endured coercive policy diffusion, where foreign actors imposed a policy course on its national government in the economic realm, when the IMF pressed for public spending cuts in the context of economic difficulties. On the other hand, in the health and social realms, the Mexican case suggests that international organisations may only hope to potentially influence domestic policymaking spaces through deliberation and learning processes. However, when faced with a populist government with a centralised and politicised response to the health crisis, as in Mexico, the possibility of developing those diffusion processes will most likely fail. Accordingly, they reveal that the contradictions and lack of coordination of global policy, as manifested in the actions of some international organisations, may act against the building up of resilient health systems.

Lastly, Heidi Smith's chapter focuses on a neglected dimension of pandemic politics: the politics of federal-state relations in Mexico during the COVID-19 pandemic. Her analysis highlights the gulf between the theory and practice of federalism during public health emergencies. She contends that Mexico's fragile federalist system was exacerbated by the COVID-19 pandemic, creating fiscal and leadership imbalances that disproportionately impacted specific states, revealing an ironic deepening of fiscal dependence on the federal government despite decentralisation efforts made since the 1980s. In Mexico, the absence of a uniform and coordinated national response to address the COVID-19 pandemic fostered a divisive politics of highly heterogeneous subnational responses among local governments whose role and capacity to carry out local public policies varied considerably. Her findings lead her to conclude that the local level is the most crucial to fighting COVID-19 in the context of a problematic federalist state, and accordingly, more attention to strengthening local institutional capacity is required.

Notes

1 On governance gaps analysis, see Weiss (2016).
2 The World Health Organization defines global public health security as "the activities required, both proactive and reactive, to minimize the danger and impact of acute public health events that endanger people's health across geographical regions and international boundaries." See www.who.int/health-topics/health-security#tab=tab_1.
3 Following Eilstrup-Sangiovanni and Westerwinter (2022, p. 237), global governance can be defined as "the process(es) whereby different types of institutions and actors, operating at different levels, and possessing different forms of authority,

exercise governance without being formally organized into a single hierarchical system of government."
4 For the original source that coined the concept of wicked problem, see Rittel and Webber (1973).

Bibliography

Aaltola, M. (2012) *Understanding the politics of pandemic scares: an introduction to global politosomatics*. London and New York: Routledge.

Aaltola, M. (2022) *Understanding the politics of pandemic emergencies in the time of COVID-19: an introduction to global politosomatics*. London and New York: Routledge.

Auld, G. *et al.* (2021) 'Managing pandemics as super wicked problems: lessons from, and for, COVID-19 and the climate crisis', *Policy Sciences*, 54, pp. 707–727.

Bayerlein, M. *et al.* (2021) 'Populism and COVID-19: how populist governments (mis)handle the pandemic', *Journal of Political Institutions and Political Economy*, 2, pp. 389–428.

Bernales-Baksai, P. and Velázquez Leyer, R. (2021) 'In search of the "authentic" universalism in Latin American healthcare: a comparison of policy architectures and outputs in Chile and Mexico', *Journal of Comparative Policy Analysis: Research and Practice*, 23(4), pp. 486–503.

Bjørkdahl, K. and Carlsen, B. (2019) *Pandemics, publics, and politics: staging responses to public health crises*. Singapore: Palgrave Pivot. https://doi.org/10.1007/978-981-13-2802-2.

Boin, A., McConnell, A. and Hart, P. (2021) *Governing the pandemic: the politics of navigating a mega-crisis*. Leiden, The Netherlands: Palgrave Macmillan. Available at: www.researchgate.net/publication/351462935_Governing_the_Pandemic_The_Politics_of_Navigating_a_Mega-Crisis.

Bringel, B. and Pleyers, G. (eds.) (2022) *Social movements and politics during COVID-19*. Bristol, UK: Bristol University Press.

Comfort, L.K. (2007) 'Crisis management in hindsight: cognition, communication, coordination and control', *Public Administration Review*, pp. 189–197.

Comfort, L.K. (2022) 'Cognition, collective action, and COVID-19: managing crises in real time', *Public Performance & Management Review*, 45(4), pp. 877–893. https://doi.org/10.1080/15309576.2022.2036204.

Comfort, L.K. *et al.* (2020) 'Crisis decision making on a global scale: transition from cognition to collective action under threat of COVID-19', *Public Administration Review*, 80(4), pp. 616–622.

Council of the Americas (2023) 'After the pandemic: considerations for COVID-19 prevention and treatment in Latin America and the Caribbean', in *AS/COA Healthcare Series*. Available at: www.as-coa.org/articles/after-pandemic-considerations-covid-19-prevention-and-treatment-latin-america-and-caribbean.

Cousins, T. *et al.* (2021) 'The changing climates of global health', *BMJ Global Health*, 6(3), pp. 1–6.

Crepaz, M. *et al.* (2022) *Viral lobbying: strategies, access and influence during the Covid-19 pandemic*. Berlin and Boston: De Gruyter.

Cyr, J. *et al.* (2021) 'Governing a pandemic: assessing the role of collaboration on Latin American responses to the COVID-19 crisis', *Journal of Politics in Latin America*, 13(3), pp. 290–236.

Daher-Nashif, S. (2021) 'In sickness and in health: the politics of public health and their implications during the COVID-19 pandemic', *Sociology Compass*, 15(6).

Davies, S.E., Kamradt-Scott, A. and Rushton, S. (2015) *Disease diplomacy: international norms and global health security*. Baltimore: John Hopkins University Press.

Davies, S.E. and Youde, J.R. (2015) *The politics of surveillance and response to disease outbreaks: the new frontier for states and non-state actors*. England: Ashgate Publishing Limited.

de Bengy Puyvallée, A. and Kittelsen, S. (2018) 'Disease knows no borders: pandemics and the politics of global health security', in Bjørkdahl, K. and Carlsen, B. (eds.) *Pandemics, publics, and politics: staging responses to public health crises*. Singapore: Palgrave Macmillan, pp. 59–73. https://doi.org/10.1007/978-981-13-2802-2_5.

De la Cerda, N. and Martínez-Gallardo, C. (2023) 'Mexico: a politically effective populist pandemic response', in Ringe, N. and Rennó, L. (eds.) *The pandemic: how populists around the world responded to COVID-19*. New York: Routledge, pp. 30–43.

Eilstrup-Sangiovanni, M. and Westerwinter, O. (2022) 'The global governance complexity cube: Varieties of institutional complexity in global governance'. *The Review of International Organizations*, 17(2), pp. 233–262.

Elbe, S. (2018) *Pandemics, pills, and politics: governing global health security*. Baltimore: Johns Hopkins University Press.

Farmer, P. (1999) 'Pathologies of power: rethinking health and human rights', *American Journal of Public Health*, 89(10), pp. 1486–1496.

Farmer, P. (2003) *Pathologies of power: health, human rights, and the new war on the poor*. Berkeley: University of California Press.

Gamlin, J. *et al.* (2021) 'Centring a critical medical anthropology of COVID-19 in global health discourse', *BMJ Global Health*, 6(6), p. e006132.

Global Health Security Index (2019) *Global health security index: building collective action and accountability*. Available at: www.ghsindex.org/wp-content/uploads/2019/10/2019-Global-Health-Security-Index.pdf.

Global Preparedness Monitoring Board (2019) *A world at risk: annual report on global preparedness for health emergencies*. Geneva: World Health Organization. Available at: www.gpmb.org/docs/librariesprovider17/default-document-library/annual-reports/gpmb-2019-annualreport-en.pdf?sfvrsn=d1c9143c_30.

Global Preparedness Monitoring Board (2020) *A world in disorder: global preparedness monitoring board annual report*. Geneva: World Health Organization. Available at: www.gpmb.org/docs/librariesprovider17/default-document-library/annual-reports/gpmb-2020-annualreport-en.pdf?sfvrsn=bd1b8933_36.

Global Preparedness Monitoring Board (2021) *From worlds apart to a world prepared: global preparedness monitoring board*. Geneva: World Health Organization. Available at: www.gpmb.org/docs/librariesprovider17/default-document-library/gpmb-annual-report-execsummary-2021.pdf?sfvrsn=b56d4ae2_48.

Gómez Dantés, O. and Frenk Mora, J. (2020) 'La pandemia y la desconfianza en la ciencia', in Senado de la República (ed.) *El mundo en tiempos de pandemia: COVID-19*. Mexico City: Instituto Belisario Domínguez, pp. 231–237. Available at: www.senado.gob.mx/64/periodico_comisionado/2020_09_el_mundo_en_tiempos_de_pandemia_COVID-19.pdf.

González Díaz, M. (2020) 'Coronavirus: health workers face violent attacks in Mexico', *BBC*, 17 May. Available at: www.bbc.com/news/world-latin-america-52676939.

Hale, T. *et al.* (2021) *Moving from words to action: identifying political barriers to pandemic preparedness*. Blavatnik School of Government, University of Oxford.

Hanson, S. and Kopstein, J. (2021) 'Understanding the global patrimonial wave', *Perspectives on Politics*, 20(1), pp. 237–249.

Hennis, A.J.M. *et al.* (2021) 'COVID-19 and inequities in the Americas: lessons learned and implications for essential health services', *Rev Panam Salud Pública*, 45. Available at: https://iris.paho.org/bitstream/handle/10665.2/55418/v45e1302021.pdf?sequence=1&isAllowed=y.

Hernández-Ruiz, L. *et al.* (2022) 'Impact of the COVID-19 pandemic on health care workers in Latin America and the Caribbean', *International Journal of Tropical Disease and Health*, 43(6), pp. 26–31.

Hoffmann, S.J. and Silverberg, S.L. (2018) 'Delays in global disease outbreak responses: lessons from H1N1, Ebola, and Zika', *AJPH Perspectives*, 108(3), pp. 329–333.

Independent Panel (2021, 2 May) *COVID-19: make it the last pandemic, the independent panel for pandemic preparedness and response.* Available at: https://theindependent-panel.org/wp-content/uploads/2021/05/COVID-19-Make-it-the-Last-Pandemic_final.pdf.

Kahl, C. and Wright, T. (2021) *Aftershocks: pandemic politics and the end of the old international order.* New York: St. Martin's Press.

Katz, R. *et al.* (2011) 'Defining health diplomacy: changing demands in the era of globalization', *The Milbank Quarterly*, 89(3), pp. 503–523.

Kushner Gadarian, S., Wallace Goodman, S. and Pepinsky, T.B. (2022) *Pandemic politics: the deadly toll of partisanship in the age of COVID.* Princeton, NJ: Princeton University Press.

Lancet Covid-19 Commission (2020) 'The lancet COVID-19 commission', *The Lancet*, 396, pp. 454–455. Available at: www.thelancet.com/pdfs/journals/lancet/PIIS0140-6736(20)31494-X.pdf.

Lasco, G. (2020) 'Medical populism and the COVID-19 pandemic', *Global Public Health*, 15(10), pp. 1417–1429.

Lasco, G. and Curato, N. (2019) 'Medical populism', *Social Science & Medicine*, 221, pp. 1–8.

Leach, M. and Tadros, M. (2014) 'Epidemics and the politics of knowledge: contested narratives in Egypt's H1N1 response', *Medical Anthropology*, 33(3), pp. 240–254.

Legler, T. (2021) 'Presidentes y orquestadores: La gobernanza de la pandemia de COVID-19 en las Américas', *Foro Internacional*, LXI(2), pp. 331–357.

Lizárraga, M.C. and Suárez, M.J. (2022) 'From "people need to hug each other, do it—and nothing will happen" to "keep a healthy distance": the Mexican government's response to the COVID-19 pandemic', in Comfort, L.K. and Rhodes, M.L. (eds.) *Global risk management: the role of collective cognition in response to COVID-19.* New York: Routledge, pp. 123–145.

Lustig, N. and Mariscal, J. (2021) 'Brazil, Mexico, and COVID-19: a striking contrast', *Journal of International Affairs*, 74(1), pp. 1–15.

Miranda, P. (2022) 'COVID-19 was the leading cause of death in Mexico in 2021', *Medscape.* Available at: www.medscape.com/viewarticle/967876.

Moreno, P. (2022) *Historias de una pandemia: El relato del infectólogo de referencia sobre el coronavirus y sus impesansables consecuencias*, Mexico City: Aguilar y Penguin Random House.

Nunes, J. (2014) 'The politics of health security', in Rushton, S. and Youde, J. (eds.) *Routledge handbook of global health security.* London: Routledge, pp. 123–134.

Ottersen, O.P. *et al.* (2014) 'The Lancet-University of Oslo commission on global governance for health: the political origins of health inequity: prospects for change', *The Lancet (Global Governance for Health)*, 383, pp. 630–667.

Palacio-Mejía, L.S. *et al.* (2022) 'Leading causes of excess mortality in Mexico during the COVID-19 pandemic 2020–2021: a death certificates study in a middle-income country', *The Lancet Regional Health—Americas*, 13, p. 100303.

Peci, A., Dussauge-Laguna, M.I. and González, C.I. (2022) 'Presidential policy narratives and the (mis)use of scientific expertise: Covid-19 policy responses in Brazil, Colombia, and Mexico', *Policy Studies*, 43(2), pp. 2–22.

Rentería, C. and Arellano-Gault, D. (2021) 'How does a populist government interpret and face a health crisis? Evidence from the Mexican populist response to COVID-19', *Brazilian Journal of Public Administration*, 55(1), pp. 1–22. Available at: www.scielo.br/j/rap/a/n39hJCcGdKzrb4Nn9M5jjjy/?lang=en.

Ringe, N. and Rennó, L. (2023) *Populists and the pandemic: how populists around the world responded to COVID-19*. London and New York: Routledge.

Rittel, H.W. and Webber, M.M. (1973) 'Dilemmas in a general theory of planning', *Policy Sciences*, 4(2), pp. 155–169.

Roberts, K.M. (2022) 'Performing crisis? Trump, populism and the GOP in the age of COVID-19', *Government and Opposition: Journal of Comparative Politics*, 57(4), pp. 1–19. https://doi.org/10.1017/gov.2022.30.

Ruckert, A. *et al.* (2016) 'Global health diplomacy: a critical review of the literature', *Social Science & Medicine*, 155, pp. 61–72.

Sánchez Talanquer, M. and Sepúlveda, J. (eds.) (2024) *Informe de la Comisión Independiente de Investigación sobre la Pandemia de Covid-19 en México*. Mexico City. Available at: www.comisioncovid.mx/.

Sánchez Talanquer, M. *et al.* (2021) *Mexico's response to COVID-19: a case study*. San Francisco: Institute for Global Health Sciences, University of California, San Francisco. Available at: https://globalhealthsciences.ucsf.edu/wp-content/uploads/2024/02/mexico -covid-19-case-study-english.pdf.

Singer, M. (2020) 'Deadly companions: COVID-19 and diabetes in Mexico', *Medical Anthropology*, 39(8), pp. 660–665. https://doi.org/10.1080/01459740.2020. 1805742.

Singer, M. *et al.* (2017) 'Syndemics and the biosocial conception of health', *The Lancet*, 389(10072), pp. 941–950. https://doi.org/10.1016/S0140-6736(17)30 003-X.

Sirleaf, J. and Clark, H. (2022) *Losing time: end this pandemic and secure the future: progress six months after the report of the independent panel for pandemic preparedness and response*. Available at: https://theindependentpanel.org/wp-content/ uploads/2021/11/COVID-19-Losing-Time_Final.pdf.

Statista Search Department (2023) *Number of novel coronavirus (COVID-19) deaths worldwide as of May 2, 2023, by country and territory* [Chart]. Statista, 2 May. www.statista.com/statistics/1093256/novel-coronavirus-2019ncov-deaths-worldwide-by-country/.

Suk, E.J. (2007) 'Sound science and the new international health regulations', *Global Health Governance*, 1(2).

Touchton, M. *et al.* (2023) 'The perilous mix of populism and pandemics: lessons from COVID-19', *Social Sciences*, 12, p. 383.

Velázquez Leyer, R. (2021) Mexico's social policy response to Covid-19: a path of minimal action. CRC 1342 Covid-19 Social Policy Response Series 5. Bremen: University of Bremen, Global Dynamics of Social Policy CRC 1342. Available at: https://media.suub.uni-bremen.de/bitstream/elib/5119/4/Mexico.pdf.

Wang, H. *et al.* (2022) 'Estimating excess mortality due to the COVID-19 pandemic: a systematic analysis of COVID-19-related mortality, 2020–21', *The Lancet*, 399, pp. 1513–1536.

Weiss, T.G. (2016) *Global governance: why? what? whither?* Cambridge, UK: Polity Press.

World Health Organization (2008) *Closing the gap in a generation: health equity through action on the social determinants of health. Final report of the commission on social determinants of health*. Geneva: World Health Organization.

World Health Organization (n.d.) 'Infodemic'. Available at: www.who.int/ health-topics/infodemic#tab=tab_1.

Ximénez-Fyvie, L.A. (2021) *Un daño irreparable. La criminal gestión de la pandemia en México*. México: Editorial Planeta.

Ximénez-Fyvie, L.A. (2022) *Las vidas que no contaron*. Mexico City: Editorial Planeta.

Zarocostas, J. (2020) 'How to fight an infodemic', *The Lancet*, 395(10225), p. 676. https://doi.org/10.1016/S0140-6736(20)30461-X.

2 Governance Gaps in Transnational Crisis Management

Mexico and WHO's Responses to COVID-19

Laura Zamudio González

Introduction

The COVID-19 pandemic represents a cross-border crisis of global proportions (Boin, McConnell and Hart, 2021, p. 10). Characterised by its severity, broad impact, rapid escalation, and the significant threat it posed to core societal values and systems, this crisis transcended geographical boundaries, political jurisdictions, and sectors. It was marked by swift, uncontrollable progression and profound uncertainty (Ansell, Boin and Keller, 2010). Given its unique nature, scale, and intensity, scholars in crisis management have labelled it a "black swan" event, an unusual, non-routine occurrence with little precedent for learning or preparation (Blondin and Boin, 2020; Boin, McConnell and Hart, 2021; Rosenthal, Hart and Charles, 1989).

The COVID-19 crisis highlighted the critical role of government responses, despite these being predominantly driven by nationalist perspectives and a tendency towards "administrative autarky" (Boin, McConnell and Hart, 2021; Michaud, 2010). This reality poses challenges to recent academic debates that emphasise the supremacy of global over local dynamics, the dispersion of authority, and the influence of private entities and transnational forces on sovereignty (Davies, Kamradt-Scott and Rushton, 2015; Stein, 2001). Similarly, assertions of an emerging post-Westphalian order, wherein non-governmental and private actors are central to defining and implementing global public policies and establishing realms of transnational administration (Moloney and Stone, 2019, p. 107; Stone and Ladi, 2015), seem less tenable considering the reassertion of states as primary crisis managers (Pierre and Peters, 2000).

Concurrently, the COVID-19 pandemic demonstrated the insufficiency of individual state efforts in addressing transnational crises (Baker and Fidler, 2006; Fidler, 2003, 2005, 2007; Novotny, 2007). In a globally interconnected context, which necessitates open information and knowledge exchange, prompt decision-making despite unclear mandates, and distributed authority, the integration of public and private resources, along with intervention strategies and mechanisms devised by international organisations, becomes imperative (Ansell, Boin and Keller, 2010; Biswas, 2021; Christensen *et al.*,

DOI: 10.4324/9781003494959-2

2016; Christensen, Laegreid and Rykkja, 2016). Although national responses often gravitated towards administrative autarky, complete isolation proved impractical for any government. To varying degrees, states were compelled to align some of their actions with global structures and actors, making the degree of coordination between national and international policies a critical factor in the governance of this transnational crisis.

Mexico, profoundly impacted by COVID-19 and experiencing significant excess mortality (UCSF, 2021), presents a stark case of pronounced political discord and minimal coordination in aligning with the strategies and positions proposed by the World Health Organization (WHO) for managing the pandemic. This chapter aims to scrutinise this discord as a manifestation of competing political interests that failed to synchronise, culminating in "governance gaps" across knowledge, policy, norms, institutions, and compliance mechanisms (Weiss, 2013). Given that the WHO is the sole international entity charged with orchestrating a response to communicable disease crises, capable of mobilising various actors and consolidating resources, this analysis focuses on how the political divergence between the Mexican government and the WHO unfolded in crisis management and the efforts of the WHO to mitigate these gaps.

This chapter endeavours to deepen the theoretical comprehension of how "governance gaps" between a nation-state and an international organisation can impede a unified response to global crises. This case is noteworthy, given the scant research on the role of international intergovernmental organisations in crisis management (Olsson and Verbeek, 2013). Literature in International Relations has primarily concentrated on the pragmatic impact of such organisations on inter-state crises (Haas, 1983) and the dysfunctions arising from their bureaucratic structures (Barnett and Finnemore, 1999, 2004). Other disciplines have explored the influence of international organisations as significant actors in global politics due to their power or authority (Avant *et al.*, 2010; Joachim, Reinalda and Verbeek, 2008; Oestreich, 2012; Reinalda and Verbeek, 1998, 2004), as well as in the contexts of global (Legler, 2013), multi-level (Bache and Flinders, 2004; Hooghe and Marks, 2003), collaborative (Ansell and Gash, 2008), indirect (Abbott and Snidal, 2010, 2015a, 2015b), and meta-governance (Sørensen and Torfing, 2009). However, there remains a substantial gap in empirical studies that elucidate organisational strategies to diminish discord in managing global crises and support the execution of essential functions such as providing meaning (a shared understanding of the nature of the threat) and control (strategies for action, methods, and rationales) (Ansell, Boin and Keller, 2010; Boin *et al.*, 2016).

The chapter is divided into three sections. The first explains the WHO's surveillance, monitoring, and response system for global crisis management. The WHO is the only international institution with an explicit mandate to contain and respond to crises caused by communicable diseases. It is also one of the few organisations to have advanced the construction of a semi-structured formal system to deal with global emergencies in which multiple actors (governmental and non-governmental) participate. The second section observes the pattern of disagreement and political discord between the Mexican government and the WHO through the identification of governance gaps, understood as institutional gaps or duplications in terms of knowledge, norms, policies, institutions, and compliance mechanisms that affected the emergence of a coordinated response and the undertaking of critical tasks for crisis management. The last section provides general reflections on Mexico's disagreement with WHO's global crisis management strategies and policies, as well as the governance procedures implemented by the WHO to encourage cooperation and close the gaps.

The WHO and Transnational Crisis Management

Crisis management, understood as the set of activities that seek to minimise the impact of the crisis on people, infrastructure, and institutions (Boin, McConnell and Hart, 2021), is an extremely complex task for governments and international organisations because, in addition to resources, it requires coordination mechanisms that encourage collective action (Boin and Bynander, 2015; Fidler, 2003; Waugh and Streib, 2006). However, the sense of urgency and uncertainty places crises in a different situation from the classic political challenges of the collective action literature (Blondin and Boin, 2020, p. 4) since it is difficult for governments to adjust preferences quickly (Boin *et al.*, 2016; Bynander and Nohrstedt, 2019). At the same time, organisations face the challenge of responding flexibly and adaptively despite having bureaucratic structures constrained by formal rules and routines (Barnett and Finnemore, 1999, 2004).

Since its creation as a specialised United Nations agency in 1948, the WHO has been tasked with addressing crises caused by communicable diseases. In the past 20 years and as a result of its intervention in the 2002 severe acute respiratory syndrome, 2009 H1NI flu, 2012 Middle East respiratory syndrome, and 2014 Ebola crises, the World Health Assembly of the organisation has broadened its mandate to include a range of events with the potential to become transnational crises, such as chemical agents and radiation, and authorised it to construct and strengthen a formal surveillance, monitoring, and response system to handle crises (Hanrieder, 2015; Kuznetsova, 2020; Taylor and Habibi, 2020).

WHO's crisis management is enshrined in the 2005 International Health Regulations (IHR) (OMS-RSI, 2008), a legally binding instrument in the field of health. In this document, the 194 member countries of the organisation delegated authority to intervene in crises caused by the emergence and expansion of infectious diseases, natural disasters, or events that have the potential to pose a threat to health security at the international level, or what the organisation describes as a Public Health Emergency of International Concern (PHEIC). PHEIC is the category whereby the WHO identifies an extraordinary event that can become a public risk for other states by spreading internationally and, therefore, requires a coordinated response (OMS-RSI, 2008, supra note 57, art. 1).

Under the IHR, the WHO will seek to *prevent, protect, contain, and control* epidemic outbreaks that threaten to spread internationally, considering that such a response is proportionate to the public health risks, while avoiding unnecessary interference in international travel and trade (OMS-RSI, 2008, Art. 2). This is a complex and to some extent contradictory mandate, as the organisation is expected to respond quickly without causing panic, efficiently without preventing the movement of people, goods, and services, and authoritatively without affecting the sovereignty of states, or becoming caught up in political interests. To fulfil this mandate, the WHO, a poorly financed organisation with an organisational structure disaggregated around six regional offices and no capacity to coerce states, experiences major challenges to conduct the surveillance, monitoring, response, and enforcement functions required by its mandate (Beigbeder, 1997; Graham, 2014; Hanrieder, 2014).

In response, the WHO has adopted a soft, indirect governance strategy known as orchestration (Abbott *et al.*, 2015a, p. 4; Hanrieder, 2015).[1] Through orchestration, the WHO links or engages, in a voluntary, non-hierarchical manner, various public and private actors who contribute resources and, acting as intermediaries, help it achieve collective objectives. From an organisational point of view, orchestration is an adaptive, low-cost strategy that offsets its lack of resources and capabilities (Dai, 2015).

The WHO's *surveillance, monitoring, and epidemic outbreak response system* is based on this practice and incorporates the work of various networks of experts, epistemic communities or knowledge networks, trans-governmental networks, private monitoring networks, foundations, companies, and non-governmental organisations (Beisheim, Campe and Schäferhoff, 2010; Haas, 1992). The WHO uses intermediaries to oversee and monitor events that could escalate into PHEIC, as well as to collect or develop scientific knowledge on such phenomena.

Surveillance, monitoring, and early warning networks enable it to identify and warn of epidemic outbreaks beyond the information provided by governments (Mykhalovskiy and Weir, 2006, p. 43; Ohrstedt *et al.*, 2018). An example of this is the Global Outbreak Alert and Response Network (GOARN), a network at the centre of the system that has become the operational arm of the WHO as it works with its Secretariat and its six regional offices.[2] GOARN makes decisions through a Steering Committee (SCOM), comprising 21 institutions and encompassing over 250 research institutes, non-governmental organisations, intergovernmental organisations, universities, and laboratories and over 600 partners worldwide.

Other networks comprising the surveillance system include the following:

- The Global Influenza Surveillance Network, which coordinates networks of laboratories and over 100 national centres specialising in flu, as well as private actors specialising in research such as the International Federation of Pharmaceutical Manufacturers and Associations, the Biomedical Advanced Research and Development Authority, the International Network of Pasteur Institutes (RIIP), and Centres of Excellence for Influenza Research and Surveillance (WHO, 2000, 2011).

- The Program for Monitoring Emerging Diseases, a public access network linking individuals who contribute to the surveillance system through email. It has 30,000 subscribers (Hugh-Jones, 2001; Madoff and Woodall, 2005; Woodall and Calisher, 2001).
- The Global Public Health Intelligence Network, a restricted access network administered by the Canadian Health Centre for Emergency Preparedness and Response.

The surveillance and monitoring efforts of the WHO, bolstered by the integration of non-governmental networks, target the initial phase of a crisis. This phase involves the early identification and declaration of an epidemiological outbreak and a PHEIC, representing the system's highest alert level (Kamradt-Scott, 2010, p. 79). During this stage, the WHO makes strategic decisions based on data from surveillance networks and epistemic communities—groups comprising experts, medical professionals, epidemiologists, virologists, and scientists associated with prominent research networks globally (Hanrieder, 2015, p. 195).

In the subsequent phase, the WHO aims to aid governments' responses by disseminating information and knowledge through various means, including protocols, technical guides, training workshops, and infographics, all designed to engender trust and enhance comprehension of the issue. It also assists in formulating response strategies and activates its coordination structures, such as the Incident Management Support Team. This team aligns the efforts of the WHO's six regional offices and 150 country offices, facilitating collaboration with governments for (i) identifying needs and (ii) preparing national response plans. In some instances, this support extends to dispatching specialised medical equipment.

However, the WHO's autonomy in surveillance and monitoring, where it has successfully implemented orchestration as a governance strategy, does not extend to response tasks. These remain the prerogative of individual states (Michaud, 2010). The IHR obligates its 194 member states to invest in developing basic response capacities, fortifying health systems, and reporting on the status of these capacities (Kluge *et al.*, 2018, p. 2). Monitoring and ensuring compliance with these tasks are conducted directly. States report to the WHO without intermediaries on their policies, and the organisation lacks peer-review mechanisms or inspection commissions to verify reported capacities (WHO, 2021, p. 4). Self-reporting of capabilities is a voluntary and discretionary act, forming the sole institutionalised mechanism for accountability.

The same happens with the WHO's recommendations to support government actions to respond to the crisis. In other words, although the IHR authorises it to issue recommendations to governments without their requesting or authorising it, the organisation lacks the legal mechanisms to enforce compliance (Fidler, 2005).

In general terms, WHO's crisis management functions are therefore punctuated by indirect governance through orchestration (in surveillance and knowledge building) and direct governance strategies (in coordinating and monitoring the response capacities of governments). The orchestration level varies and has not been institutionalised in all the response stages and functions. Insofar as the response system falls to governments and the WHO has failed to promote intermediaries to pressure for the adoption of policies or strengthen their response capacities and lacks direct enforcement mechanisms, one challenge for the WHO is to ensure that the convergence of interests emerges not as the result of a deliberate attempt to create or impose hierarchical order but through the progressive establishment of a semi-structured system of orchestration that will permit, facilitate, or encourage the enlistment of multiple actors through the convergence of knowledge, norms, and institutions (Boin and Bynander, 2015; Olsson and Verbeek, 2013, p. 329).

This institutional architecture for managing transnational crises shows that the WHO contemplates several governance strategies to exercise its surveillance, monitoring, coordinating, and response functions. Orchestration is the key strategy for overcoming its organisational limits. The following section analyses the way this system and the various forms of governance interacted in the Mexican government's handling of COVID-19.

Governance Gaps in Crisis Management Between Mexico and the WHO

In recent years, the WHO expanded its crisis management mandate and advanced in the construction of a surveillance, monitoring, coordination, and response system, addressing the five functions considered critical for crisis management: early warning, creation of meaning, horizontal and vertical coordination, strategic decisions, and learning (Blondin and Boin, 2020). Theoretically, these functions encourage the creation of a culture of surveillance and permanent monitoring with mechanisms for the communication and transmission of knowledge that enable collective understanding of the nature, characteristics, and potential effects of the threat, as well as a roadmap on what to do, how, and why.

However, cooperation between international actors and organisations in contexts of anarchy and collective stress is not automatic (Rosenthal, Hart and Charles, 1989). The existence of an institutional structure to provide a formal response is important, but since there is no global government with centralised, hierarchical control mechanisms, the interaction of actors with diverse interests and objectives opens knowledge, policy, regulatory, institutional, and compliance gaps that influence and tend to fragment collaborative management of the crisis.

Governance gaps, understood as omissions or inconsistencies, spaces or areas where actions and fundamental tasks are required to achieve order, stability, and predictability (Weiss, 2013, p. 128), constitute a useful analytical instrument for analysing problems and challenges in the coordination of responses between the Mexican government and the WHO. Knowledge gaps refer, for example, to the lack of shared understanding among actors about the nature, causes, severity, and magnitude of a problem. This gap explains the way knowledge is produced, questioned, and challenged, because although the production of knowledge, data, and scientific evidence is subject to the visions of groups of experts and epistemic communities, they interact with politicians and public officials in various parts of the world, hindering the common, consensual understanding of an issue (Coronado, 2021).

This shared understanding constitutes one of five areas of the pandemic politics literature identified in the introduction to this volume, termed symbolic politics, which observes the political element in responses to public health emergencies of international concern (Bjorkdahl and Carlsen, 2019; Davies and Youde, 2015; Bengy and Kittelsen, 2019). Specifically, symbolic politics consists of the construction of a collective cognition, or the framing of a situation, in this case, of a public health problem recognised as a threat. It is the creation of a shared vision among the various actors involved in the response process constructed through political communication processes.

Failure to bridge a knowledge gap has implications for standards and policies since both elements also require a certain level of consensus and consistency between the international and the domestic (Weiss, 2013, p. 129).

Norms are defined as behaviour patterns that are commonly accepted and involve processes of collective approval or disapproval (Weiss, 2013, p. 134). They undergo processes of socialisation and internalisation until they are accepted as appropriate behaviour, exempt from questioning by governments and citizens (Finnemore and Sikkink, 1998), and are perceived based on the way an accepted behaviour is framed. When governments need to justify behaviour that is not in line with the norm, this indicates that the norm exists and that they recognise they are failing to abide by it.

Policies, understood as the interrelated set of government objectives and principles as well as agreed programmes of action and implementation to achieve those principles, may lead to the paralysis or aggravation of any crisis. International organisations are places where states codify norms and transform them into global policies (Weiss, 2013, p. 141). However, international organisations and officials lack the resources and mechanisms to implement them, creating a significant disconnection from or inconsistency with states, which remain the relevant political authorities. Furthermore, policies do not exist in a vacuum; they are embodied in institutions, which ideally have resources and autonomy. Institutional gaps therefore refer both to gaps in legal matters (codified rules) and norms and to formal structures (organisations) that help coordinate collective decision-making processes (Weiss, 2013, p. 145).

Lastly, the compliance gap highlights the political will to provide resources, since, without it, implementation, monitoring, and enforcement problems arise. In general terms, there is a lack of compliance mechanisms at the international level, and the strategy of "naming and shaming" is often used, which occurs when organisations publicly demonstrate mismanagement of an issue. The strategy of "naming and shaming" is one of the most important for enforcing compliance (Weiss, 2013, p. 155).

On the basis of this analytical framework, it is immediately clear that the case of Mexico shows a situation of disagreement, the result of governance gaps in all areas of interaction, with significant impacts on the possibilities of organisation and coordination.

That said, we can see that in the case of Mexico, the knowledge gap was extremely pronounced and prevented a shared understanding of the nature and severity of the phenomenon. The conceptualisation of the threat, risk level, and response time were out of step and completely different for Mexico and the WHO. In terms of *pandemic politics*, the symbolic politics between these two entities differed regarding the severity of the threat, the temporality, and the measures to be taken. While WHO's actions were governed and modified according to the available scientific research of the international community, in Mexico, decisions were more relaxed, and both the recognition and responses to the emergency on the part of the authorities took place late, regarding the former.

The WHO Expert Committee, tasked with verifying and reporting the severity of a threat, classified COVID-19 as a serious disease and categorised it as a PHEIC on January 30, 2020. Its first recommendations were undoubtedly contradictory and hinted at a certain optimism about the early possibilities of breaking the chain of contagion through collective action. The declaration of a pandemic on March 11, 2020, however, revealed the weak reaction of governments to the declaration of a PHEIC and the organisational inability to develop a global response. As the WHO acquired information from the scientific community, research networks, and epistemic communities, it was able to support governments with strategic plans—such as the Strategic Preparedness and Response Plan and the Global Humanitarian Response Plan COVID-19—designed to identify needs, provide technical and logistical support, send specialised medical equipment, disseminate information, practices, and general recommendations on the clinical management of the virus, the use of face masks, mass diagnostic testing, identification measures, and tracing and isolation (WHO, 2020a, 2020b). Consulting with networks and epistemic communities also forced the WHO to be flexible and change the course of action or correct its approaches in response to the emergence of new scientific evidence, as happened when a group of scientists asked it to reconsider the issue of aerial transmission of the virus in closed spaces (Mandavilli, 2020; Morawska and Milton, 2020).

In Mexico, the political authorities responsible for managing the crisis claimed that COVID-19 was a disease of "low virulence compared to influenza" (Sotomayor, 2020; UCSF, 2021). They systematically dismissed the recommendations issued by the scientific community, such as the use of face masks and the usefulness of mass testing, and spread misinformation based on incomplete statistics and inadequate surveillance systems on the evolution of contagions or the null possibilities of contagion of asymptomatic people (Erdely, 2020; Ornelas-Aguirre and Vidal-Gómez, 2020).[3] The most important response measures to combat COVID-19—National Social Distancing, the Marine Plan, and the DN-III Plan—were launched late, two months after the WHO had declared a PHEIC and almost a month after the first contagion had been registered in the country (Cruz Reyes and Patiño Fierro, 2021). Official recognition of a "serious priority disease" was not announced until March 31, when the country shifted from phase I, characterised by "external or exported contagion," to phase II of "local transmission," with over a thousand confirmed cases. This behaviour links directly to the policy area of compliance and implementation of the International Health Regulations 2005, within the *pandemic politics* literature (Davies and Youde, 2015), which notes that moments lacking conclusive evidence or certainty about disease severity are exploited in political terms by governments to delay compliance measures.

The knowledge gap regarding COVID-19 contrasts with the Mexican government's response to H1N1 in 2009. Since Mexico was the epicentre of the pandemic, the problem was perceived as serious, an immediate reaction was elicited, and coordination with the WHO was sought. Only three days after the first cases were identified, a pandemic alert was issued, and ten days later, a national emergency was declared (Córdova-Villalobos *et al.*, 2009, p. 2). Following the pandemic alert, all activities in federal public administration (except strategic activities), mass public events, and classes throughout the country were suspended.[4] In addition, Mexico sought regional coordination with its main trading partners, the United States and Canada, and sent virus samples to the US Centers for Disease Controland Prevention and the Winnipeg Laboratory in Canada (Córdova-Villalobos *et al.*, 2009, p. 2; Hernández-Ávila and Alpuche-Aranda, 2020).

The disparity in the perceptions of the threat and the sense of urgency between Mexico and the WHO to overcome COVID-19 negatively affected the collaborative handling of the crisis. The discrepancy was public since, on several occasions, the WHO has questioned the Ministry of Health of the Mexican government about its attitude towards COVID-19 (Sotomayor, 2020), calling for the authorities to "take the pandemic seriously" (Morán, 2020). Various media, inside and outside the country, have noted the lack of flexibility of the authorities in modifying their position, ignoring internationally recognised scientific evidence and information, as happened with the proven importance of increasing the number of tests to contain the spread of the virus.[5]

The political and institutional gaps highlight the way Mexico and the WHO formulated and implemented actions and mobilised resources for dealing with COVID-19. WHO's strategic decisions and policy formulation are based on a universalist conception, which abstracts particularisms, which have been highlighted and studied in the literature as a pathology or organisational dysfunction (Barnett and Finnemore, 1999). However, despite this, countries adopted or adapted some WHO's recommendations to control the acute stage of the pandemic. Southeast Asian countries, for example, adopted the proposal to identify, trace, and isolate cases, applying sophisticated tracking technologies and mechanisms, while others acted contrary to the IHR by closing borders and preventing the flow of goods and people. In short, the basic WHO's recommendations for pandemic control were (i) containment (breaking the chain of contagion); (ii) early identification (mass testing); (iii) tracing (surveillance and monitoring); and (iv) isolation of cases.

In Mexico, strategic decisions were affected by the complex economy versus health dilemma. Certainly, the economy had been stagnant since the third quarter of 2018 (Martínez, Torres and Orozco, 2020, p. 10), with poverty levels of 49.5%, equivalent to 61.7 million people (CONEVAL, 2018). However, the impossibility of adjusting national policies to WHO's recommendations can be explained largely by populism, a policy of fiscal austerity, and the government's priority to continue with costly construction projects such as the Tren Maya, the Felipe Angeles International Airport, and the Dos Bocas refinery (Cruz Reyes and Patiño Fierro, 2021, p. 35). This situation explains (although it does not justify) that instead of containment, the government has adopted a mitigation policy with a low economic cost, which resulted in the refusal to apply massive tests for early identification of cases or, in the decision to lift the only national confinement that, for a month and a week, suspended all non-essential economic activities as well as face-to-face education, just when the contagions began to increase (Ximénez-Fyvie, 2021, p. 96; UCSF, 2021, p. 59). For most of the pandemic, isolation and quarantine policies were voluntary, justified on the grounds of the defence of human rights and freedoms. Advocacy, however, was not accompanied by significant economic support from the federal government for economically vulnerable individuals and groups. As an ECLAC study shows, the fiscal and social protection response in Mexico was the most limited within Latin American countries and the world (Blofield, Giambruno and Filgueira, 2020). Mexico would also be the only country that would not implement support measures to address the social and economic deterioration of the pandemic in the migrant population (Vera-Espinoza *et al.*, 2020), even though the WHO urged governments to aid migrants, stateless persons, internally displaced persons, and refugees.[6]

Contrasting sharply with the WHO's political-strategic focus on containment policies such as active surveillance, early detection, isolation, case management, and contact tracing, Mexico opted for mitigation strategies. These were "epidemiologically" rationalised based on the perceived inevitability of the pandemic and a miscalculated belief that promoting widespread infection would lead to a form of "herd immunity" (Sotomayor, 2020; Ximénez-Fyvie,

2021, p. 96; UCSF, 2021, p. 59). Politically, this approach manifested in a form of medical populism (Lasco and Curato, 2019), characterised by entrusting doctors, particularly public officials under presidential command, to lead the response. This stance positioned them against independent experts and specialists who questioned the scientific validity of governmental decisions (Renteria and Arellano-Gault, 2020, p. 175). Moreover, these officials often openly questioned the scientific information provided by the international community and the WHO specifically.

This medical populism is indicative of a broader political strategy, marked by centralised and discretionary decision-making subordinated to the executive branch (UCSF, 2021, p. 55). Despite constitutional mandates assigned to the General Health Council, the highest health policy collegiate body with decision-making authority during health emergencies, it was sidelined. The president delegated the responsibility of directing the pandemic response to the Undersecretariat of Prevention and Health Promotion, a unit within the Secretariat of Health directly under presidential control. This crisis management model resulted in policies being determined by a group of officials politically and administratively subordinate to the president without input or scrutiny from independent technical experts (UCSF, 2021, p. 55).

This governance model facilitated discretionary decision-making steeped in political motivations, eschewing scientific deliberation and obstructing coordination with pivotal stakeholders (UCSF, 2021, p. 57). Notably, it overlooked insights from Mexican chemist and Nobel Laureate Mario Molina regarding the airborne transmission of the virus (Morawska and Milton, 2020; Zhang *et al.*, 2020). Similarly, it disregarded the recommendations of former health secretaries advocating for an increase in testing and a unified coordination strategy nationwide (Chertorivski *et al.*, 2020; Vera, 2020). This approach culminated in dire outcomes, including the highest global mortality rate of healthcare workers due to COVID-19 by year's end. The president's actions, which often contradicted WHO's guidelines on mask-wearing and social distancing, not only downplayed the gravity of the emergency but also projected a narrative of inconsistency and neglect towards the nation's commitments.

The influence of the executive was further exemplified by the involvement of the armed forces. While the Mexican military has a long-standing tradition of aiding civilians in disasters and emergencies, and their participation through Plan Marina and DN-III was crucial in addressing the crisis—providing specialised medical staff, activating military hospital units, managing voluntary isolation centres, ensuring hospital security, and handling the transportation and storage of supplies, among other tasks (Cruz Reyes and Patiño Fierro, 2021, p. 20)—a political undertone was evident in the management of these efforts.

The normative gap was also present in the interaction between the responses of Mexico and the WHO. Pandemic containment is a global norm derived from the IHR, and the different warnings from the WHO about the mismanagement of the pandemic in Mexico should be understood as a mechanism of "shaming" or "embarrassment," due to its non-compliance with the norm. According to the IHR, states acquire the obligation to adopt structural and capacity-building measures that will contribute to the objective of *preventing, protecting, controlling, and providing a public health response to the spread of a disease* (WHO, 2005). Article 5 establishes that each state must develop, strengthen, and maintain the capacity to detect, manage, notify, and report IHR-related events and respond in a timely, effective manner to public health risks and emergencies of international concern (WHO, 2005). At the national level, preparedness measures include the establishment and operation of an emergency response plan with containment and control mechanisms and the establishment of a national IHR liaison body (WHO, 2005).

In this respect, Mexico submitted a report on its capacities to the WHO in 2020, and it acknowledged that its response capacity to zoonotic events was below the world average (WHO, 2021). The percentage for other indicators was as follows: 100% in coordination with IHR, focal point, and with the surveillance system; 87% in national emergency structure and provision of health services; 80% in legislation and financing, human resources, food safety, risk communication, points of entry, chemical events, and radiation emergencies (WHO, 2020a). Unfortunately, these indicators did not effectively translate into pandemic management, which would invite a review of the indicators analysed and their veracity.

The compliance gap was also noticeable since the WHO lacks mechanisms to enforce compliance. It does not have peer-review mechanisms, nor is it authorised to send on-site inspection and verification teams, as the International Atomic Energy Agency does, to determine whether the capacity reports submitted by states reflect the actual situation (Bartolini, 2021; Gostin, Moon and Mason, 2020).

The interaction between the Mexican government and the WHO for dealing with the pandemic therefore reveals governance gaps in all areas. This shows that the actors failed to harmonise their interests or reach a consensus on the nature of the problem or the control mechanisms, especially the WHO's recommendations regarding mass testing, case tracking and monitoring, and the emphasis on containment rather than mitigation.

The disagreement between Mexico and the WHO was not absolute. Mexico did join the COVID-19 Tools (ACT) Accelerator, the time-limited interagency coordination initiative promoted by WHO to socialise the cost and economic risk in the research and development of treatments and vaccines (Eccleston-Turner and Upton, 2021, p. 427). With an economic contribution of US$850,000, out of a basket of US$17.9 billion (SRE, 2020), Mexico was admitted to the COVAX facility, one of the four pillars of the accelerator, and purchased 51.1 million doses to immunise 25.75 million people, as well as joining the vaccine production circuits (SRE, 2021a, 2021b).[7] The COVAX facility is financed with donations from rich countries and advance purchases of vaccines to encourage laboratories and research centres to invest and research diagnostic tests, effective treatments, and vaccines. COVAX promised to offer vaccines at affordable prices to cover 20% of the population of each country. From a governance point of view, the accelerator demonstrates the ability to mobilise networks (Lee and Piper, 2020).

Other initiatives implemented by the WHO, which sought to establish semi-structured spaces for collaboration, included, for example, the development and free distribution throughout Latin America of Go. Data, a type of software for tracking and monitoring cases during epidemic outbreaks[8], and the electronic platforms—COVID-19 Partners Platform[9], COVID-19 Intra-action Review, COVID-19 Supply Chain Network[10], WHO (COVID-19) Disease Dashboard, etc.—designed to support governments in their purchase, logistics and financial resources, in addition to linking them directly with foundations, laboratories, and companies.

The disparity between the political interests and interpretations regarding COVID-19 and the urgency of responses made the challenge of collective coordination extremely complex. The WHO cannot impose itself on governments, but they require information, knowledge, and collective cost-sharing mechanisms to deal with transnational crises. Thus, navigating a worldwide health crisis in the absence of coordination mechanisms and instruments with global actors with no coordination between policies, rules, and knowledge also affects the real possibilities of domestic control.

Mexico was one of the countries most affected by COVID-19 and one of the countries with the highest excess mortality (El Informador, 2022; UCSF, 2021). Various analysts maintain that COVID-19 could never be controlled, meaning that Mexicans did not experience the process in waves with clearly identified peaks and troughs and instead remained in a situation in which it was not possible to "flatten the curve." The lack of coordination with the WHO's crisis management system does not fully explain this situation because, in addition to the economic problems, the Mexican population suffered from pre-existing health problems such as obesity, diabetes, and other chronic diseases that aggravated cases. However, the discrepancy between the WHO and its epistemic networks also affected domestic governance.

Final Thoughts

It would seem evident that to address transnational health crises like COVID-19, governments would be willing to coordinate not only with internal actors but also with external ones. It would seem logical that to strengthen their response capacity to the crisis, they would be open to receiving information, knowledge, assistance, and resources from multiple actors, especially from international organisations understood as impartial, technocratic, and specialised entities. However, the case presented in this chapter shows that this was not necessarily the case.

The relationship between the Mexican government and the WHO in managing the pandemic shows that what ultimately prevailed was a pattern of political disagreement, characterised by distrust, questioning, and permanent confrontation. Thus, instead of reaching a shared understanding of the crisis (its nature, severity, dimensions, etc.) and of the possible actions to control it, the Mexican government politicised its relationship with the WHO—branding it as intrusive and an instrument of the great powers—hindering reasonable minimum collaboration and eluding the logics of governance based on knowledge and the best information available. Governments are not obliged to adopt WHO's recommendations. The International Health Regulations only commit them to report annually on the state of their response capacities, alert a possible international public health emergency, and not to close borders or obstruct the exchange of goods and services in an emergency context. However, the rejection by the Mexican government was so visible and obstinate that it even ventilated a national policy full of false and pseudoscientific epidemiological arguments, which continue to be questioned by the expert community both inside and outside the country. Despite the scientific evidence and better understanding of the virus that developed over time, in Mexico, these explanations were neither accepted nor did they alter the course agreed upon for the management of the pandemic, resulting in a huge number of deaths.

Populist governments often distrust technical experts, question the validity and neutrality of scientific information, and attack international organisations for their intrusive tendencies. And certainly, organisations are not neutral actors, devoid of agency; they have interests, define their tasks, and adopt strategies that were not previously agreed upon by states. They offer interpretations, propose tasks that correspond to their technical expertise, and present themselves as apolitical actors without necessarily being so. While the populist reaction of a country like Mexico is not necessarily the fault of an organisation like the WHO, however, one thing is clear: In the face of the populist onslaught that many countries in the world are suffering, international organisations need to adapt their discourses and strategies. How then could an organisation like the WHO support the response to the pandemic crisis when, de facto, it is rejected by populist governments?

The governance gaps reviewed in this chapter, specifically knowledge, policy, and institutional gaps, highlight the fact that the Mexican government deliberately sought to position itself against the WHO to strengthen arguments for internal political control. These governance gaps did not allow for the creation of mechanisms, policies, tasks, and actions to reduce uncertainty. Without a common understanding of the problem and a shared sense of the threat, it was not possible to outline a roadmap and pool efforts, assign tasks, and share costs to control the phenomenon.

The failure to achieve a common understanding of the problem led the Mexican government to reject many of the policies and recommendations of the WHO aimed at containing the virus and breaking the chain of transmission. Instead of containing the virus spread through early detection mechanisms such as mass testing, distancing and mask-wearing, surveillance, monitoring, and confinement proposed by the WHO, a mitigation policy was adopted that left the population to resolve many of the dilemmas imposed by the pandemic on its own. Mitigation was a less costly policy (economically) as it avoided investment in mass COVID-19 detection tests or terms of prolonged confinement, but it was politically advantageous as it positioned the government in a different argumentative position, centred on the idea that contagion was inevitable and that it was necessary to wait until "herd immunity" was reached. Unfortunately, this epidemiological approach had net negative effects and led to the country not "flattening the curve" of infections, resulting in tens of thousands of preventable deaths. However, the government achieved its objective: to continue polarising society and undermining various institutional logics of checks and balances, all to stay in power.

Although the information provided by the WHO cannot be considered neutral and apolitical, various political calculations led the WHO to take different decision-making channels and policies in a situation of emergency and high uncertainty. This meant that at various times it was also not able to provide consistent and accurate information. What is certain is that the WHO was able to provide information coming from specialised instances, inhabited by doctors, epidemiologists, and pandemic experts. It is also true that, with its flaws, it provided information and proposed policies based on the learning of the network of organisations and governments around the world. The WHO is, with all its flaws and limitations, a space for linking hundreds of scientists working in research institutes, public and private laboratories, and organisations with economic and technological resources to propose responses in an open and transparent manner. From the WHO, very important information was launched about the nature of contagions, training was offered through online workshops, specialised protocols were developed for health service personnel, infographics for the population, monitoring platforms, donor platforms, and platforms to access markets. The monitoring and tracking of the pandemic, as well as the transparent and open movement of information, allowed for adjusting policies and reviewing decisions.

In Mexico, decisions were taken within a small group of public officials and medical officials who rejected the evidence and were absolutely unwilling to change their decisions so as not to contradict the country's president. They politicised their positions, rejecting information coming from independent doctors and experts, preferring to feed their own ambitions. With this centralised decision-making model, the institutional governance gap with the WHO was also widened.

In cases of crisis, the WHO activates an incident management mechanism with contacts at regional and national levels. Through contact points, the WHO usually helps in identifying needs, resources, and essential mechanisms to prevent the collapse of health systems and design response plans. As such, the WHO does not have the capacity to respond for governments but can complement and strengthen their response through information, logistical support, access routes to markets for scarce goods, linking with donors, direct assistance from foreign doctors, as well as creating coalitions and resource pools to address the phenomenon and mitigate its effects on vulnerable populations.

Populist governments tend to politically exploit attacks on expert knowledge to strengthen their political goals of control, in this case, for example, through exaggerating arguments in defence of national sovereignty. This argument limits possibilities for collaboration and coordination and attempts to ensure impunity and little accountability for the real effects caused by an emergency. In Mexico, the presence of the armed forces also played a role in the centralisation and control of decision-making and coordination mechanisms. Indeed, the armed forces often play a key role in managing emergencies such as earthquakes or floods, so it is not surprising that they were at the forefront of the response. However, what should be studied is the way in which the army also affected coordination with PAHO and WHO.

In summary, the case demonstrates that there were governance gaps between the Mexican government and the WHO. The government rejected the organisation's interpretations and recommendations for managing the pandemic, enduring public controversy in order to position itself politically and justify its increasingly centralised decisions that strengthened executive power.

On a positive note, it can be observed that the WHO has made notable gains in global cooperation mechanisms like the Vaccine Accelerator and COVAX. These initiatives were innovative, showcasing WHO's historic ability to rally governments and various actors in temporary, horizontal, and semi-structured collaborative frameworks. For instance, COVAX is a coalition of actors co-led by CEPI, Gavi, and the WHO, with UNICEF playing the role of the implementing actor. Furthermore, WHO plays a critical role in managing vaccine distribution through its Global Allocation Framework. This framework aids governments in developing national vaccination strategies and infrastructure. It utilises tools such as the COVID-19 Vaccine Introduction Readiness Tool and the VIRAT Dashboard Platforms, along with the PAHO Regional Platform for Access to Innovation for Health Technology. Similarly, the Health Connector, a joint venture led by Unitaid, the Wellcome Trust, the Global Fund, the World Bank, and the WHO and supported by the Global Financing Facility for Women, Children, and Adolescents, serves to highlight WHO's commanding presence in regulatory policy (WHO, 2021, p. 6).

The WHO demonstrated a capacity that extends beyond its technical expertise: the ability to foster cooperation among countries, private organisations, and academic communities through soft governance strategies known as orchestration. This approach has historically been successful in pooling resources and forming coalitions with diverse stakeholders. Through these methods, the WHO encourages collaboration among actors in a decentralised and horizontal fashion, without prominent or obvious hierarchies. The participation of the Mexican government in these initiatives raises important questions. Could these horizontal action frameworks be more resilient to politicisation and challenges from populist governments? Do they provide more cost-effective coordination strategies for governments when interacting with external actors? Furthermore, the pandemic has underscored the necessity for international organisations to re-evaluate the foundations of their legitimacy in an increasingly politically polarised world. In such a context, neutrality or mere expertise alone is insufficient. There is a growing need to emphasise the value of knowledge, transparency, and more horizontal forms of governance to effectively address international challenges.

Notes

1 This behaviour is not exclusive to the WHO; many organisations address complex problems by developing inter-organisational cooperation strategies through dyads, triads, or specific fields (Biermann and Harsch, 2017; Koops, 2017), hybrid structures (Abbott and Faude, 2021; Cornforth and Spear, 2010), nested structures (Blavoukos and Bourantonis, 2017), and meta-organisations (Ahrne and Brunsson, 2005), among many other forms of action.

2 The regional areas of GOARN include the following: the Americas Regional Office (AMRO), comprising 14 partners and eight networks; the Africa Regional Office (AFRO), with eight partners and four networks; the Eastern Mediterranean Regional Office (EMRO), with six partners and three networks; the European Regional Office (EURO), with 61 partners and 17 networks; the South-East Asian Regional Office (SEARO), with 14 partners and three networks; and the Western Pacific Regional (WPRO), with 50 partners and five networks (Mackenzie *et al.*, 2018).

3 This happened with the "Sentinel" surveillance model that provides estimates and general figures of infected people with severe symptoms who are admitted to hospitals yet proved unsuitable for detecting new diseases such as COVID-19, with high rates of asymptomatic cases (Ramírez, 2020).

4 Contrary to 2020, these measures were delayed, and in fact various states such as Jalisco, Guanajuato, Yucatán, Michoacán, Tamaulipas, Sonora, Nuevo León, Tlaxcala, Colima, and Veracruz unilaterally cancelled classes and began to implement their own response actions (Cejudo, 2020; Cejudo *et al.*, 2020).

5 Only 39 tests were performed per thousand people nationwide during the first year of the pandemic (UCSF, 2021, p. 86; Hellewell *et al.*, 2020; Liang *et al.*, 2020).

6 Mexico, together with Argentina, Bolivia, Brazil, Chile, Colombia, Costa Rica, the Dominican Republic, Ecuador, Panama, Paraguay, Peru, Trinidad and Tobago, and Uruguay, was considered a country affected by the Venezuelan refugee crisis and entered the humanitarian response plan that contemplated helping 4.5 million migrants and displaced persons (WHO, 2020a, pp. 29–32; ONU México, 2020).

7 Mexico has received and packaged over 60 million doses since the start of the pandemic, and it is estimated that this figure will have reached 70 million by mid-July, which has made it possible to send vaccines, produced in collaboration with Argentina, to Paraguay, Belize, Bolivia, El Salvador, Honduras, Guatemala, and Jamaica. Packaging has been conducted at the Drugmex plant in Querétaro, Liomont Laboratories in the State of Mexico, and the state-owned Birmex has started packaging tests for the Russian Sputnik V vaccine (SRE, 2021a).

8 For further information, see www.who.int/godata. Mexico joined this initiative in March 2020, through a workshop for health officials www.paho.org/es/noticias/2-3-2020-inician-mexico-puesta-marcha-godata-america-latina-tool-to-investigate-0.
9 Platform comprising 120 countries and 80 donors that evaluates the implementation of the response pillars as well as the financial or technical needs of countries.
10 Portal for the supply market that linked commercial agencies and supply centres for respirators and protective equipment.

References

Abbott, K. and Faude, B. (2021) 'Hybrid institutional complexes in global governance', *The Review of International Organizations*.

Abbott, K. and Snidal, D. (2010) 'International regulation without international government: improving IO performance through orchestration', *Review of International Organizations*, 5, pp. 315–344.

Abbott, K. *et al.* (2015a) *International organizations as orchestrators*. Cambridge: Cambridge University Press.

Abbott, K. *et al.* (2015b) 'Two logics of indirect governance: delegation and orchestration', *British Journal of Political Science*, 46(4), pp. 719–729.

Ahrne, G. and Brunsson, N. (2005) 'Organizations and meta-organizations', *Scandinavian Journal of Management*, 21(4), pp. 429–449.

Ansell, C., Boin, A. and Keller, A. (2010) 'Managing transboundary crises: identifying the building blocks of an effective response system', *Journal of Contingencies and Crisis Management*, 18(4), pp. 195–207.

Ansell, C. and Gash, A. (2008) 'Collaborative governance in theory and practice', *Journal of Public Administration Research and Theory*, 18, pp. 543–571.

Avant, D. *et al.* (eds.) (2010) *Who governs the globe?* Cambridge: Cambridge University Press.

Bache, I. and Flinders, M. (eds.) (2004) *Multi-level governance*. Oxford: Oxford University Press.

Baker, M.G. and Fidler, D. (2006) 'Global public health surveillance under new international health regulations', *Emerging Infectious Diseases*, 12(1), pp. 1058–1065.

Barnett, M. and Finnemore, M. (1999) 'The politics, power, and pathologies of international organizations', *International Organization*, 53(4), pp. 699–732.

Barnett, M. and Finnemore, M. (2004) *Rules for the world: international organizations in global politics*. USA: Cornell University Press.

Bartolini, G. (2021) 'The failure of "core capacities" under the WHO international health regulations', *International and Comparative Law Quarterly*, 70, pp. 23–250.

Beigbeder, Y. (1997) *The internal management of United Nations organizations: the long quest for reform*. New York: St. Martin's Press.

Beisheim, M., Campe, S. and Schäferhoff, M. (2010) 'Global governance through public-private partnerships', in Enderlein, H., Wälti, S. and Zürn, M. (eds.) *Handbook on multi-level governance*. UK: Edward Elgar Publishing Limited.

Bengy, P. and Kittelsen, S. (2019) 'Disease knows no borders: pandemics and the politics of global health security', in Bjørkdahl, K. and Carlsen, B. (eds.) *Pandemics, publics, and politics*. Singapore: Palgrave Pivot.

Biermann, R. and Harsch, M. (2017) 'Resource dependence theory', in Biermann, R. and Joachim, A.K. (eds.) *Palgrave handbook of inter-organizational relations in world politics*. UK: Palgrave MacMillan, pp. 135–157.

Biswas, S. (2021) 'The coronavirus pandemic and global governance: the domestic diffusion of health norms in global health security crises', *Jadavpur Journal of International Relations*, 25(2), pp. 208–234.

Bjorkdahl, K. and Carlsen, B. (eds.) (2019) *Pandemics, publics, and politics*. Singapore: Palgrave Pivot.

Blavoukos, S. and Bourantonis, D. (2017) 'Nested institutions', in Biermann, R. and Joachim, A.K. (eds.) *Palgrave handbook of inter-organizational relations in world politics*. UK: Palgrave MacMillan, pp. 303–319.

Blofield, M., Giambruno, C. and Filgueira, F. (2020, September) 'Policy expansion in compressed time: assessing the speed, breadth and sufficiency of post COVID-19 social protection measures in 10 Latin American countries', *CEPAL, Social Policy*, 235.

Blondin, D. and Boin, A. (2020) 'Cooperation in the face of transboundary crisis: a framework for analysis', *Perspectives on Public Management and Governance*, 20(20), pp. 1–13.

Boin, A. and Bynander, F. (2015) 'Explaining success and failure in crisis coordination', *Geografiska Annaler: Physical Geography*, 97(1), pp. 123–135.

Boin, A., McConnell, A. and Hart, P. (2021) *Governing the pandemic: the politics of navigating a mega-crisis*. Leiden, The Netherlands: Palgrave McMillan.

Boin, A. *et al.* (2016) *The politics of crisis management: public leadership under pressure*. Cambridge: Cambridge University Press.

Bynander, F. and Nohrstedt, D. (2019) *Collaborative crisis management: inter-organizational approaches to extreme events*. London and New York: Routledge.

Cejudo, G. (2020) 'Alianza federalista: cronología de un desencuentro', *Nexos*, 5 November.

Cejudo, G. *et al.* (2020) *Federalismo en COVID: ¿Cómo responden los gobiernos estatales a la pandemia?* México: CIDE.

Chertorivski, S. *et al.* (2020) *La gestion de la pandemia en México. Análisis preliminar y recomendaciones urgentes*. Mexico: Consejo consultivo ciudadano.

Christensen, T., Laegreid, P. and Rykkja, L.H. (2016) 'Organizing for crisis management: building governance capacity and legitimacy', *Public Administration Review*, 76(6), pp. 887–897.

Christensen, T. *et al.* (2016) 'Comparing coordination structures for crisis management in six countries', *Public Administration*, 94(2), pp. 316–332.

CONEVAL (2018) 'Resultados de pobreza en México 2018 a nivel nacional y por entidades federativas'. [Online]. Available at: www.coneval.org.mx/Medicion/MP/Paginas/Pobreza-2018.aspx (Accessed 13 January 2024).

Córdova-Villalobos, J.A. *et al.* (2009) 'The influenza A (H1N1) epidemic in Mexico. Lessons learned', *Health Research Policy Systems*, 7(21). [Online]. Available at: www.health-policy-systems.com/content/7/1/21 (Accessed 13 January 2024).

Cornforth, C. and Spear, R. (2010) 'The governance of hybrid organizations', in Billis, D. (ed.) *Hybrid organizations in the third sector: challenges of practice, policy and theory*. Basingstoke: Palgrave.

Coronado, M.E. (2021) 'La gobernanza global de la salud y los límites de las redes de expertos en la respuesta al brote de la COVID-19 en México', *Foro Internacional*, 2(244), pp. 469–505.

Cruz Reyes, G. and Patiño Fierro, M.P. (2021) 'Las medidas del Gobierno Federal contra el virus SARS-CoV2 (COVID-19)', *Cuaderno de Investigación*, 6. DGDyP/IBD.

Dai, X. (2015) 'Orchestrating monitoring: the optimal adaptation of international organizations', in Abbott, K.W., Genschell, P. and Snidal, D. (eds.) *International organizations as orchestrators*. Cambridge, UK: Cambridge University Press, pp. 134–165.

Davies, S.E., Kamradt-Scott, A. and Rushton, S. (2015) *Disease diplomacy: international norms and global health security*. Baltimore, MD: John Hopkins University Press.

Davies, S.E. and Youde, J.R. (2015) *The politics of surveillance and response to disease outbreaks: the new frontier for states and non-state actors*. London and New York: Routledge.

Eccleston-Turner, M. and Upton, H. (2021) 'International collaboration to ensure equitable access to vaccines for COVID-19: the ACT-accelerator and the COVAX facility', *The Milbank Quarterly*, 29(2), pp. 426–449.

El Informador (2022) 'COVID: México, primer lugar en índice de muertos por coronavirus', *3 de enero 2022*. [Online]. Available at: www.informador.mx/mexico/COVID-Mexico-primer-lugar-en-indice-de-muertos-por-coronavirus-20220103-0096.html (Accessed 14 January 2024).

Erdely, A. (2020) 'Algunas dudas sobre la aritmética de la secretaría de Salud', *Nexos*, 20 abril. [Online]. Available at: www.nexos.com.mx/?p=47756 (Accessed 14 January 2024).

Fidler, D. (2003) 'Disease and globalized anarchy: theoretical perspectives on the pursuit of global health', *Social Theory Health*, 1, pp. 21–41.

Fidler, D. (2005) 'From international sanitary conventions to global health security: the new international health regulations', *Chinese Journal of International Law*, 4(2), pp. 325–392.

Fidler, D. (2007) 'SARS: political pathology of the first post-Westphalian pathogen', *Journal of Law, Medicine & Ethics*, 31(4), pp. 485–505.

Finnemore, M. and Sikkink, K. (1998) 'International norm dynamics and political change', *International Organization*, 52(4), pp. 887–917.

Gostin, L., Moon, S. and Mason, B. (2020) 'Reimagining global health governance in the age of COVID-19', *AJPH Reimagining Public Health*, 110(11), pp. 1615–1619.

Graham, E. (2014) 'International organizations as collective agents: fragmentation and the limit of principal control at the World Health Organization', *European Journal of International Relations*, 20(2), pp. 366–390.

Haas, E. (1983) 'Regime decay: conflict management and international organizations 1945–81', *International Organization*, 37(2), pp. 361–380.

Haas, P. (1992) 'Introduction: epistemic communities and international policy coordination', *International Organization*, 46(1), pp. 1–35.

Hanrieder, T. (2014) 'The path-dependent design of international organizations: federalism in the World Health Organization', *European Journal of International Relations*, 21(1), pp. 215–239.

Hanrieder, T. (2015) 'WHO orchestrates? Coping with competitors in global health', in Abbott, K. *et al.* (eds.) *International organizations as orchestrators*. Cambridge: Cambridge University Press, pp. 191–213.

Hellewell, J. *et al.* (2020, 28 February) 'Feasibility of controlling COVID-19 outbreaks by isolation of cases and contacts', *Lancet*, 8(4).

Hernández-Ávila, M. and Alpuche-Aranda, C.M. (2020) 'Mexico: lessons learned from the 2009 pandemic that help us fight COVID-19', *Healthcare Management Forum*, 33(4), pp. 158–163.

Hooghe, L. and Marks, G. (2003) 'Unravelling the central state, but how? Types of multi-level governance', *American Political Science Review*, 97(2), pp. 233–243.

Hugh-Jones, M. (2001) 'Global awareness of disease outbreaks: the experience of ProMED-mail', *Public Health Reports*, 116(Supplement 2), pp. 27–31.

Joachim, J., Reinalda, B. and Verbeek, B. (2008) *International organizations and implementation: enforcers, managers, authorities?* London and New York: Routledge.

Kamradt-Scott, A. (2010) 'The WHO secretariat, norm entrepreneurship and global disease outbreak control', *Journal of International Organizations Studies*, 1(1), pp. 72–89.

Kluge, H. *et al.* (2018) 'Strengthening global health security by embedding the international health regulations requirements into national health systems', *BMJ Global Health*, pp. 1–7. [Online]. https://doi.org/10.1136/bmjgh-2017-000656 (Accessed 14 January 2024).

Koops, J. (2017) 'Inter-organizationalism in international relations: a multilevel framework of analysis', in Biermann, R. and Koops, J. (eds.) *Palgrave handbook of inter-organizational relations in world politics*. UK: Palgrave MacMillan, pp. 189–217.

Kuznetsova, L. (2020) 'COVID-19: the world community expects the World Health Organization to play a stronger leadership and coordination role in pandemics control', *Frontiers in Public Health*, 8.

Lasco, G. and Curato, N. (2019) 'Medical populism', *Social Science & Medicine*, 221.

Lee, K. and Piper, J. (2020) 'The WHO and the COVID-19 pandemic', *Global Governance*, 26, pp. 523–533.

Legler, T. (2013) 'Gobernanza global', in Legler, T., Santa Cruz, A. and Zamudio, L. (eds.) *Introducción a las Relaciones Internacionales: América Latina y la Política Global*. Mexico: Oxford University Press, pp. 253–266.

Liang, L.-L. *et al.* (2020) 'COVID-19 mortality is negatively associated with test number and government effectiveness', *Scientific Reports*, 10(12567).

Mackenzie, J. *et al.* (2018) 'The global outbreak alert and response network', *Global Public Health*, 9(9), pp. 1023–1039.

Madoff, L. and Woodall, J.P. (2005) 'The internet and the global monitoring of emerging diseases: lessons from the first 10 years of ProMED-mail', *Archives of Medical Research*, 36(6), pp. 724–730.

Mandavilli, A. (2020) 'WHO: to review evidence of airborne transmission of coronavirus', *The New York Times*, 7 July.

Martínez, J., Torres, M.C. and Orozco, E.D. (2020, March) *Características, medidas de política pública y riesgos de la pandemia del COVID-19*. Senado de la República: Instituto Belisario Dóminguez.

Michaud, J. (2010) 'Governance implications of emerging infectious disease surveillance and response as global public goods', *Global Health Governance*, 3(2), pp. 1–16.

Moloney, K. and Stone, D. (2019) 'Beyond the state: global policy and transnational administration', *International Review of Public Policy*, 1(1), pp. 104–118.

Morán, C. (2020) 'La OMS llama la atención de México y Brasil por el curso de la pandemia', *El País*, 30 November. [Online]. Available at: https://elpais.com/mexico/sociedad/2020-11-30/la-oms-llama-la-atencion-a-mexico-y-brasil-por-el-curso-de-la-pandemia.html (Accessed 3 and 13 January 2024).

Morawska, L. and Milton, D.K. (2020) 'It is time to address airborne transmission of coronavirus disease 2019 (COVID-19)', *Clinical Infectious Diseases*, 71(9), pp. 2311–2313.

Mykhalovskiy, E. and Weir, L. (2006) 'The global public health intelligence network and early warning outbreak detection', *Canadian Journal of Public Health*, 97(1), pp. 42–44.

Novotny, T. (2007) 'Global governance and public health security in 21st century', *California Western International Law Journal*, 38(6), pp. 19–40.

Oestreich, J. (2012) *International organizations as self-directed actors. A framework for analysis*. London and New York: Routledge.

Ohrstedt, D. *et al.* (2018) 'Managing crises collaboratively: prospect and problems—a systematic literature review', *Perspectives on Public Management and Governance*, 1(4), pp. 257–71.

Olsson, E.-K. and Verbeek, B. (2013) 'International organizations and crisis management', in Reinalda, B. (ed.) *Routledge handbook of international organization*. London and New York: Routledge, pp. 324–336.

ONU México (2020) *ONU necesita 350 millones de dólares para el plan de respuesta humanitaria contra el coronavirus*. Información Oficial de las Naciones Unidas. [Online]. Available at: https://coronavirus.onu.org.mx/la-onu-necesita-350-millones-de-dolares-para-el-plan-de-respuesta-humanitaria-contra-el-corona virus (Accessed 15 November 2023).

Ornelas-Aguirre, J.M. and Vidal-Gómez Alcalá, A. (2020) 'Crítica al modelo centinela de vigilancia epidemiológica en la COVID-19', *Cirugía y Cirujanos*, 88(6), pp. 753–764.

Pierre, J. and Peters, G. (2000) *Governance, politics and the state.* New York: St. Martin´s Press.

Ramírez, S. (2020, 9 April) 'Centinela: qué es, por qué no es (necesariamente) ideal para COVID-19 y pues, ahora qué', in *Mexicanos contra la corrupción y la impunidad.* [Online]. Available at: https://contralacorrupcion.mx/modelo-centinela-que-es-COVID-19/ (Accessed 10 January 2024).

Reinalda, B. and Verbeek, B. (1998) *Autonomous policy making by international organizations.* London and New York: Routledge.

Reinalda, B. and Verbeek, B. (eds.) (2004) *Decision making within international organizations.* London and New York: Routledge.

Renteria, C. and Arellano-Gault, D. (2020) 'How does a populist government interpret and face a health crisis? Evidence from Mexican populist response to COVID-19', *RAP Brazilian Journal of Public Administration*, 55(1), pp. 169–185. https://doi.org/10.1590/0034-761220200524.

Rosenthal, U., Hart, P. and Charles, M.T. (1989) 'The world of crises and crisis management', in Rosenthal, U., Hart, P. and Charles, M.T. (eds.) *Coping with crises: the management of disasters, riots and terrorism.* Springfield, IL: Charles C. Thomas Publishers, pp. 3–36.

Sørensen, E. and Torfing, J. (2009) 'Making governance networks effective and democratic through metagovernance', *Public Administration*, 87, pp. 234–258.

Sotomayor, G. (2020) 'La OMS corrige a la Secretaría de Salud por su reacción al coronavirus', *Revista Proceso*, 2 March. [Online]. Available at: www.proceso.com.mx/reportajes/2020/3/2/la-oms-corrige-la-secretaria-de-salud-por-su-reaccion-al-coron avirus-239300.html (Accessed 14 January 2024).

SRE (2020) 'México participará en COVAX Facility para la obtención de vacunas contra COVID'19', *Comunicado 256*, 7 September. Available at: www.gob.mx/sre/prensa/mexico-participara-en-covax-facility-para-la-obtencion-de-vacunas-contra-COVID-19.

SRE (2021a) 'México, entre los 10 primeros lugares en abastecimiento de vacunas gracias a la estrategia de diversificación y envasado en el país', *Comunicado 312*, 13 July.

SRE (2021b) 'Gracias al envasado en México, se ha acelerado el abasto de vacunas contra COVID'19', 14 July. [Online]. Available at: www.gob.mx/sre/es/articulos/gracias-al-envasado-en-mexico-se-ha-acelerado-el-abasto-de-vacunas-contra-COVID-19–277252?idiom=es (Accessed 14 January 2024).

Stein, A. (2001) 'Constrained sovereignty. The growth of international intrusiveness', in Rosecrance, R. (ed.) *The new great power coalition: toward a world concert of nations.* New York: Rowman & Littlefield Publishers Inc, pp. 261–281.

Stone, D. and Ladi, S. (2015) 'Global public policy and transnational administration', *Public Administration*, 93(4), pp. 839–855.

Taylor, A. and Habibi, R. (2020) 'The collapse of global cooperation under the WHO international health regulations at the outset of COVID-19: sculpting the future of global health governance', *American Society of International Law Insights*, 24(5). [Online]. Available at: www.asil.org/insights/volume/24/issue/15/collapse-global-cooperation-under-who-international-health-regulations (Accessed 14 January 2024).

UCSF. (2021) *La respuesta de México al COVID-19: Estudio de Caso.* Institute for Global Health Sciences.

Vera, R. (2020) 'Exsecretarios de Salud urgen al gobierno a cambiar la estrategia contra el COVID-19', *Revista Proceso*, 9 September.

Vera-Espinoza, M. *et al.* (2020) 'Towards a typology of social protection for migrants and refugees in Latin America during the COVID-19 pandemic', *Comparative Migration Studies*, 9(52). https://doi.org/10.1186/s40878-021-00265-x.

Waugh, W. and Streib, G. (2006) 'Collaboration and leadership for effective emergency management', *Public Administration Review*, 66, pp. 131–140.

Weiss, T. (2013) *Global governance. What? Why? Whither?* Cambridge, UK: Polity Press.

WHO (World Health Organization) (2000, 26–28 April) 'Global outbreak alert and response', in *Report of a WHO meeting*. Geneva, Switzerland: World Health Organization. WHO/CDS/CSR/2000.3. Unpublished document.

WHO (World Health Organization) (2005) *International Healt Regultions*. Geneva. Switzerland: World Health Organization.

WHO (World Health Organization) (2011; 30 November to 3 December 2010) 'Strengthening the WHO global influenza surveillance network (GISN)', in *Report of the 3rd meeting with national influenza centers (NICs) held in Hammamet*. Geneva, Tunisia: World Health Organization. [Online]. Available at: www.who.int/influenza/gisrs_laboratory/GISN_Meeting_Report_apr2011 (Accessed 14 January 2024).

WHO (World Health Organization) (2020a, April–December) *Global humanitarian response plan COVID-19*. United Nations Coordinated Appeal.

WHO (World Health Organization) (2020b, 3 February) *Novel coronavirus (2019-nCov): strategic preparedness and response plan*. Geneva, Switzerland: World Health Organization.

WHO (World Health Organization) (2021, 12 January) *Strengthening preparedness for health emergencies: implementation of the international health regulations (2005)*. Geneva: Executive Board EB148/19.

Woodall, J. and Calisher, C. (2001) 'ProMED-mail: background and purpose', *Emerging Infectious Diseases*, 7(3), p. 563.

Ximénez-Fyvie, L.A. (2021) *Un daño irreparable. La criminal gestión de la pandemia en México*. México: Editorial Planeta.

Zhang, R. *et al.* (2020) 'Identifying airborne transmission as the dominant route for the spread of COVID-19', *Proceedings of the National Academy of Sciences*, 117(26).

3 Rethinking the Role of Epistemic Communities in the International Response to Pandemics

Mexico's Response to COVID-19[1]

María Esther Coronado Martínez

Introduction

Pandemic responses require an efficient provision of global public goods through collective action with high levels of cooperation. With this goal, the current system of global health governance (reformed after the outbreak of SARS in 2003) has tried to implement changes for better international pandemic preparedness and response. The updated International Health Regulations (IHR) (WHO, 2008) approved by the World Health Assembly in 2005 are at the centre of this system. Although the revised 2005 IHR brought a more coherent approach, the governance system is still fragmented, with severe gaps and deficiencies that hinder a coordinated and efficient response to COVID-19 (WHO, 2021c).

The 2005 IHR was, for the first time, implemented in 2009 to respond to the H1N1 influenza pandemic. Since then, the regulations have shown their limitations. With COVID-19, the international response exposed severe constraints in a poorly coordinated, disjointed global system with many national and individual responses.

International relations scholars have tried to explain why and how global problems such as pandemics shape international cooperation. Their research has yielded a set of theoretical and empirical concepts based on global governance, where different actors and mechanisms participate, such as international organisations, networks of professionals, and non-governmental organisations (NGOs), among others (Deacon, 2007; Haas, 1992; Jenson, 2010; Ruggie, 1998). Embedded in the fundamentals of global governance, transnational administration closely analyses how these actors are involved in the global policy process and its implementation (Legrand, 2015; Stone and Ladi, 2015).

Embedded in these theoretical concepts, this chapter presents an analysis of the role of epistemic communities and their engagement in the international dissemination of ideas in the case of Mexico's response to the COVID-19 pandemic. The central argument considers that pandemics' global health governance system has configured various epistemic communities as dissemination mechanisms of ideas based on scientific evidence. They promote cooperation

DOI: 10.4324/9781003494959-3

and collaboration to respond to pandemics and implement agreements and standards created within the World Health Organization (WHO), such as the 2005 IHR. These groups can influence the implementation of global policies through their specialised experience and knowledge, helping to justify and support decisions made at the national level (evidence-based policy), partly due to their members' position in the policymaking process at the national and global levels. Their influence, however, is inconsistent and difficult to predict since their connection to this process is not always clear. Additionally, they are not isolated from political influence (Legrand, 2015; Sending, 2019; Spath, 2005), which affects their legitimacy.

This analysis explores why epistemic communities have failed to disseminate global policy recommendations to manage the COVID-19 pandemic. It hypothesises that although central in the decision-making process during the COVID-19 emergency, epistemic communities have had to contend with the increased politicisation of some of their key members, causing weaknesses and fractures in their networks' internal structures and thus affecting their ability to promote the adoption of global recommendations at the national level. As this book underscores, these actors were not isolated from political influence and, in cases like Mexico, contributed to constructing a narrative where politics and personal agendas downplayed the risk of the outbreak.

The first part of the chapter introduces the analytical framework to examine the research question. It presents a model to operationalise epistemic communities as a causal mechanism that influences decision-making to understand how politics comes into play. The second section discusses epistemic communities and the participation of transnational networks in global health. The third section explores the case of Mexico and the response to COVID-19 as a test case of the theoretical framework, a methodology commonly used in epistemic community theory (Alexander and Bennett, 2005; Davis Cross, 2013; Haas, 2015, p. 7; Karlsson, 2004). The last section offers concluding remarks.

Theoretical Framework: Global Governance and Expert Networks

Within constructivism, knowledge is a variable that affects state behaviour (Haas, 2004). Collective action at the international level results from the different learning processes and how states adopt and use policy models (Kurowska and Kratochwill, 2012; Haas, 2004; Underdal, 1998). Governments will adopt and implement internationally prescribed policies to the extent that they are compelling models for powerful actors and can persuade others (Wendt, 1992; Weyland, 2006). There is an interaction between policy diffusion, policy convergence, and the dissemination of ideas. Policy diffusion explains which policies, institutions, and ideas of a particular political system are adopted in another political system (Stone, 2008) and communicated through specific channels (Berry and Berry, 2007; Stone, 2012). Policy convergence facilitates the adoption and implementation of international actions. States may adopt and implement internationally prescribed policies when these alternatives have previously worked somewhere else under similar circumstances (Berry and Berry, 2007; Stone, 2012; Wendt, 1992; Weyland, 2006). Dissemination of ideas implies a transfer by which certain institutions, policies, or knowledge (applied at one time and/or place) are used to develop institutions or policies elsewhere (Dolowitz and Marsh, 1996; Evans, 2004; Stone, 2012).

In this context, global governance is defined as a set of arrangements adopted by state and non-state actors to promote collective action, achieve a common goal, and produce public goods to solve global problems (Dodgson and Lee, 2002; Frenk and Moon, 2013; Zacher and Keefe, 2007). Therefore, global governance is "a layered and complex system of independent and interdependent ideas, interests, institutions, actors, movements, and relations that perform governance functions" (Lennox, 2008, p. 7).

Under this non-traditional paradigm of the international system, the process of global politics, rather than the nation-state, is the independent variable of study (Stone and Ladi, 2015, p. 852). The role of international organisations as makers of ideas, political networks, and, in general, non-state actors is essential in shaping results (Deacon, 2007; Haas, 1992; Haas, 2015; Jenson, 2010). These actors' interactions are central to learning and influence (Lennox, 2008). The global governance system provides an arena where technical and efficient solutions are sought, leaving aside politics and focusing on common solutions that benefit all people (Spath, 2005, p. 38). Policy outcomes are based on information, knowledge, and ideas (Haas, 1992; Haas, 2004), while transfer occurs at a broader level via different routes, such as expert networks (Stone, 2012, p. 485). Therefore, the construction of policies based on scientific evidence and experts within the global governance system is crucial to efficiently implementing policies that address problems in specific fields.

Among these groups of experts, the epistemic community stands out, defined as "a network of professionals, from a variety of disciplines and backgrounds, with recognised experience and competence in a particular area and who are considered policy-relevant authorities within that domain or subject area" (Haas, 1992, p. 3). Epistemic communities are networks of professionals and experts in a specific field of policy/knowledge (Haas, 1992). These professionals share notions of validity, a common language and culture (Morin, 2014), normative beliefs, causal beliefs, epistemological criteria, and a mutual understanding of policies (Haas, 1992). They connect actors and transmit information (Karlsson, 2004; Keck and Sikkink, 1999), create inter-organisational alliances, and promote broad bonds among their members. These experts connect with NGOs, governments, international organisations and their secretariats, epistemic communities in other fields and levels (national and international), and different types of networks. Their ideas are transferred through international working groups, committees, or expert groups (Karlsson, 2004; Stone, 2012).

The assumptions behind the theoretical concept of epistemic communities, however, tend to be challenged by academics. Critics of epistemic communities argue that without a clear definition of the causal mechanism that makes it possible to influence the policymaking process, it is hard to agree that these groups are responsible for successful cooperation outcomes. Besides, other elements are ignored, such as policymakers' absolute demand for knowledge (Dunlop, 2009; Löblová, 2018) and the epistemic community's capacity to bargain and build alliances necessary for disseminating its ideas (Sebenius, 1992; Zito, 2018). To deal with this problem, scholars have proposed approaches such as distinguishing between external and internal characteristics (Ribhi Shawar, 2016), clearly defining a causal mechanism (Löblová, 2018, p. 161), and applying concepts of social network theory to explain specific attributes of these actors (Petersen, 2016). In addition to the problems with the methodology, a considerable number of researchers apply this approach only to successful cases (Davis Cross, 2013; Dunlop, 2009; Löblová, 2018), and the identification of an epistemic community is not always clear since its definition is interpreted narrowly, referring most of the time only to scientists and technicians (Davis Cross, 2013; Morin, 2014), without identifying who the members are (Coronado, 2019) or their roles in the community.

To address these issues, first, it is central to understand the causal mechanism described in Haas' definition to address these methodological and empirical problems. According to Löblová (2018), Haas' concept has four main components: (1) the emergence of a group of experts (the epistemic community itself); (2) the pursuit of a policy goal that will be achieved through the dissemination of knowledge; (3) its members' level of "penetration" in decision-making structures to influence from within and their access to spaces that allow them to influence policymakers to adopt the epistemic community's knowledge and interpretation of the problem/solutions; and (4) the cost-benefit analysis made by decision-makers to adopt or not the epistemic community's preferences (Löblová, 2018, pp. 164–165). The first two elements in this mechanism are the foundation of any epistemic community and correspond to its internal structure. The other two elements depend on external components since epistemic communities are embedded in the international system where international organisations and national governments are still the main actors (see Figure 3.1). The combination and interaction of these characteristics will translate into the epistemic community's ability to influence international cooperation, which this research defines as the ability to convince a government to adopt global policies and recommendations to address the COVID-19 pandemic (Coronado, 2019). Nonetheless, this mechanism does not automatically lead to success and can be disrupted and

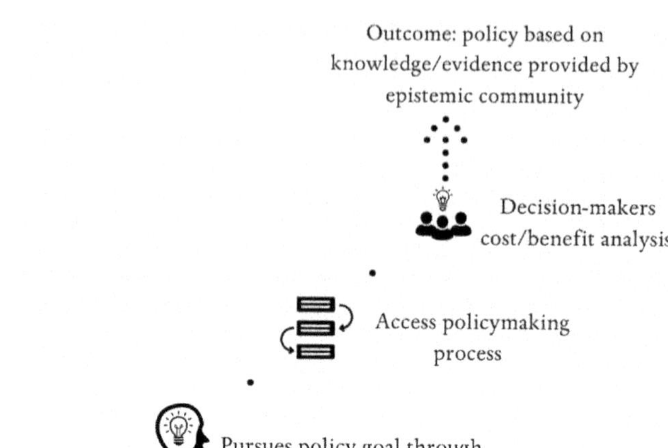

Figure 3.1 Epistemic communities' causal mechanism, created by the author based on Haas (1992) and Löblová (2018)

influenced by internal or external elements. Hence, an epistemic community's success will depend on factors found in this process.

Second, it is essential to recognise the epistemic community's members and, as a group, how its internal characteristics are essential to its level of success and its connections to other networks. In this regard, this research broadens the definition, referring to an "epistemic community network" as one or more groups of professionals embedded in the system of global health governance, connecting and interrelating its members through their common interest and understanding of a particular problem, sharing epistemological beliefs and principles (Coronado, 2019). For an epistemic community network to exist, its members should share consensual knowledge (Haas, 1992; Hasenclever, 2000; Karlsson, 2004), leading to an informed joint action that can alter perceptions of the area of possible agreement (Haas, 1992; Sebenius, 1992). Once it has been possible to generate consensual and usable knowledge about the policy problem and its possible solutions, it can be transmitted to decision-makers. As a network and cohesive group, the epistemic community affects the perceived area of a possible arrangement in that all members agree on the issue (Adler and Haas, 1992; Karlsson, 2004; Sebenius, 1992).

However, since knowledge is constantly disputed, disagreements are common among experts. These disagreements can create rivalry within the network and other expert groups (Antoniades, 2003; Morin, 2014, p. 280). Rivalry influences policymaking, as contested knowledge is difficult to translate into clear policies or actions (Haas, 2004; Morin, 2014; Youde, 2005). In addition, the divergences among experts can affect the legitimacy of the decisions that derive from them since there will be more questioning about the transparency and legitimacy of the decision-making process.

The epistemic community must have consistent beliefs and a policy project that resonates with other experts and people in general (Sebenius, 1992, p. 360). The power to persuade policymakers to adopt specific knowledge requires the epistemic community to show solid internal cohesion and professionalism. Internal cohesion provides the group with an episteme, a shared worldview derived from mutual socialisation and knowledge (Davis Cross, 2013, p. 147). The greater the homogeneity in values, perspectives, and sense of mission, the lower the conflict of interest. These characteristics also make it less complicated for expert groups to reach and maintain agreements on the actions or policies that are most appropriate to solve a specific problem (Davis Cross, 2013; Sebenius, 1992), allowing them to build a common policy objective and influence the policy process to achieve it.

Epistemic community networks can influence international and domestic processes by shaping the interests and behaviour of other actors (Antoniades, 2003; Davis Cross, 2013). Experts can shape the political debate, providing justifications for alternatives and catalysing national or international coalitions in supporting selected policies and advocating for change (Weiss, Carayannis and Jolly, 2009). Therefore, they can "change the game" to set up possible solutions and bring states closer to the ideal outcome (Sebenius, 1992). The ability of experts to position themselves as authorities on the subject and to be heard by decision-makers assumes that these groups of experts have some degree of power in world politics (Antoniades, 2003, p. 21; Haas, 2004; Sebenius, 1992). Power and knowledge are generally competitive alternatives (Sebenius, 1992). However, knowledge is power, and expert groups can control it. Scientifically supported decisions may reflect hidden values as science incorporates implicit values that symbolise power and dominance (Haas, 2004).

The methodological complexity of the epistemic community concept requires thinking about it in a broader context. Transnational management proposes notions that connect the epistemic community network and its methods to mobilise and transform their expertise into policy outcomes. In this conceptualisation, global governance is an administrative action that focuses on the policymaking process rather than politics (Sending, 2019, p. 389). Governments engage in transnational administration when faced with problems of a global nature, where expert networks are essential to address these problems (Legrand, 2015, p. 206). This notion considers how global public policies are regulated, managed, and implemented by actors operating beyond the borders and jurisdiction of the nation-state (Legrand, 2015, p. 840). Hence, it identifies transgovernmental networks as groups of experts and decision-makers who can mobilise resources and power within their territories (Legrand, 2019, p. 205), connected through a communication network that facilitates the transfer of ideas. Transgovernmental networks have direct access to information and influence the decision-making process. They have direct contact with their peers nationally and internationally and collaborate across formal and informal methods to solve collective problems (Legrand, 2019, p. 201; Raustiala, 2002, p. 1).

Transnational networks help to reduce the space between governments and international organisations, serving as a bridge in the governance system (Legrand, 2019, p. 212). Furthermore, they are instruments for exchanging ideas and information and coordinating policies without resorting to more formal mechanisms (Legrand, 2019, p. 212). They are experts in a field that spatially goes beyond traditional borders and can have normative objectives and values in common (Sending, 2019, p. 389). These networks have been essential for the influence of international organisations, either as members or as connecting gear to the governance system (Keohane and Nye, 1974, p. 55). Nonetheless, they can bring other problems since their informality leads to a lack of transparency and public participation with limited legitimacy in a democratic system (Skogstad, 2003).

In practice, epistemic community networks include different groups or subgroups of experts that align themselves around an identified policy outcome and analyse it from different perspectives. Since the conceptual lines separating the epistemic community from a trans-governmental network are vague, this research integrates transgovernmental networks with the epistemic community network, especially in areas that need a high level of expertise and knowledge for decision-making (see Figure 3.2).

The connection between epistemic communities and transgovernmental networks links the former directly with domestic politics. Epistemic community networks can influence the policy process due to the position of their members: as bureaucrats, diplomats, or national and international policymakers (Antoniades, 2003; Davis Cross, 2013; Sebenius, 1992). Their position also permits the consolidation of bureaucratic power and, within this, the ability to institutionalise their influence and insert their point of view within the political process, increasing the likelihood that their ideas will be disseminated and adopted in the decision-making process (Antoniades, 2003, p. 32; Haas, 1992; Sending, 2019). Though it is not always clear how epistemic community members' position warrants their influence, linking transgovernmental networks as a subgroup of epistemic community networks opens a space for the latter and connects them directly to the policy process. In this sense, epistemic community members who are part of a transgovernmental network have more possibilities to influence the global policy process and adopt global policies at the national level.

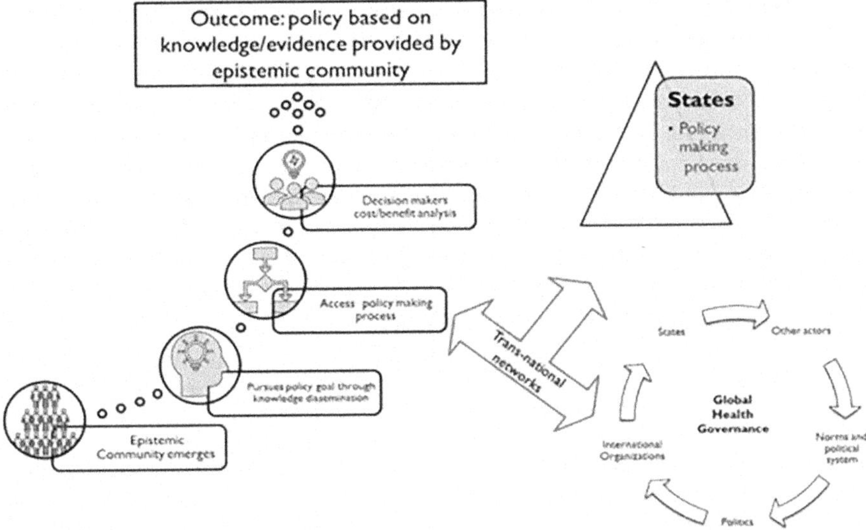

Figure 3.2 Relationship epistemic communities and transgovernmental networks

Source: Author's design

This connection, however, makes epistemic communities more susceptible to political influences and interference, affecting their position as
knowledge authorities since their performance in the global governance
system is not independent of the dynamics of the nation-state. Although
power and knowledge are generally treated as competitive alternatives and
science and politics observe different principles, when epistemic community
networks claim their role as authorities in an area of knowledge, they exercise a type of power (Majone, 1989, p. 3; Sebenius, 1992). Therefore, the
distributive consequences of science-based advice can be political (Haas,
2004), which occurs in negotiations with political actors and governments,
resulting in politics overshadowing scientific evidence (Cozzens and Woodhouse, 1995).

During the COVID-19 outbreak, it is possible to identify how these
factors have affected epistemic community networks. There have been differences within the international epistemic community network between
those experts working with the WHO and those not directly affiliated with
it. For instance, although airborne transmission of the virus was finally
recognised as the primary method of contagion, it took some time to create
policies adopting this evidence. In April 2020, experts in the field of "aerosol science" held a videoconference with Michael Ryan, head of the WHO's
Health Emergencies Programme, and Maria Van Kerkhove, technical lead

of the WHO's COVID-19 response, and the Infection Prevention and Control Guidance Development Group (IPC GDG) (an expert group advising the WHO on infection containment; Lewis, 2022, p. 27). The expert group led by Lidia Morawska, an aerosol scientist at the Queensland University of Technology in Brisbane, Australia, presented the WHO's expert group with evidence of aerosol transmission (Lewis, 2022, p. 26). However, after this meeting, the WHO did not change its recommendations. Given that the IPC GDG did not agree with this suggestion, in July 2020, 239 scientists published a request to change the international strategy. They presented clear evidence of contagion through the aerosol effect in enclosed spaces. They asked the WHO to accentuate measures to mitigate transmission by these means, providing evidence that demonstrated COVID-19 was spreading by air (Morawska and Milton, 2020). This public call for action was aimed at the WHO to review the evidence and modify its recommendations (Mandavilli, 2020). In August 2020, experts from the IPC GDG published a document stating that "Based on the scientific evidence accumulated to date, our view is that SARS-CoV-2 is not spread by the airborne route to any significant extent" (Conly *et al.,* 2020, p. 1). The expert group collaborating with the WHO was not convinced that the evidence was conclusive enough to prove this type of transmission (Conly *et al.,* 2020). The WHO gradually changed its perspective and introduced the term "airborne transmission for COVID-19" in 2021 (Lewis, 2022).

In the case of political influence, the pandemic has exacerbated people's dissatisfaction with science and the evidence it produces, driven partly by the *infodemic* during the pandemic. Some governments ignored evidence-based recommendations, constraining the dissemination of experts' advice (Fleming, 2020; Horton, 2020). For instance, since the beginning of the epidemic in Brazil, national experts from the epistemic community faced challenges in implementing measures that originated at the global level. Former health ministers Luiz Henrique Mandetta (January 2019–April 2020) and Nelson Teich (April–May 2020) defended applying measures based on scientific evidence, confronting President Jair Bolsonaro's stance on minimising the pandemic. Even though the former ministers were direct members of a transgovernmental network and the epistemic community, with the possibility of influencing decision-making to disseminate global policies, their recommendations were ultimately not accepted by the head of state, and they resigned from their positions (Hallal, 2021).

In the United States, something similar happened within the relationship between former President Donald Trump (2017–2021) and the scientists who made up the White House's Coronavirus Task Force. There were signs of disagreement early in the pandemic, especially with the group's leader, Anthony Fauci (Behrmann and Santucci, 2020). The latter, a renowned expert in infectious diseases with a very close link to the global epistemic community, was often questioned by the president for endorsing guidelines derived from an international consensus but which did not resonate with the political interests of the then-president (Niel, 2021). Divergent perspectives ultimately caused Fauci to be often relegated and ignored, creating divisions among the country's experts that affected the ability of the national epistemic community to influence policy. In this instance, the experts' ability to disseminate and transmit policies was reduced since evidence-based recommendations from the global community did not resonate with political interests (Stevens, 2007).

In Mexico, the central case in this research, adopting global policies transmitted and disseminated through the epistemic community network encountered similar problems. This argument will be expanded in the following sections.

Global Health Governance and Expert Networks in the Pandemic Response

Global health assumes that most public health problems are interdependent and must be addressed globally (Dodgson and Lee, 2002; Fidler, 2010; Frenk and Moon, 2013; Zacher and Keefe, 2007). In this system, international institutions and norms are instrumental in creating a system of governance that aims to reach and protect people worldwide (Lee and Fidler, 2007; Youde, 2011). The current global health system has the WHO at its core. The organisation has worked as a technical actor to build an international consensus on global health policy. It creates and disseminates guidelines and standards, engaging expert groups and committees to produce evidence-based knowledge. With these mechanisms, the WHO becomes a connector of experts, establishing and coordinating epistemic communities and trans-governmental networks in different spheres of global health (Culebro, 2020).

Coordinating global public health measures is necessary for effective international responses to pandemics. The 2005 IHR provides agreed guidelines for that aim. In the process, experts become indispensable in applying the regulations that consolidate the definition of policies arising from global health governance. Experts with diverse backgrounds (diplomats, politicians, bureaucrats, scientists, epidemiologists, among others) and from different nationalities confirm outbreaks, carry out surveillance, investigate cases, collect data, identify the population at risk through contact tracing, identify pathogens, develop therapies, and apply control and prevention measures (Condon and Patel, 2006; Kamradt-Scott, 2013; McKee, Gilmore and Schwalbe, 2005; World Health Organization, 2000). All of these are necessary steps to manage and respond to a pandemic.

Although the 2005 IHR does not explicitly mention networks of experts as actors, it allocates a primary role to them (World Health Organization, 2008) and their advice. Scientific evidence is thus essential to support the implementation of the IHR during a pandemic.[2] For instance, Article 12 of the 2005 IHR defines an Emergency Committee (EC) as the central technical entity for assessing an outbreak. The EC has an advisory role to the Director General (DG) of WHO and will recommend whether an event should be declared a Public Health Emergency of International Importance (PHEIC). It also states that the WHO and its DG should consider scientific principles, available scientific evidence, and information for all different response components when assessing an outbreak. Article 47 stipulates that the DG must establish a "Roster of Experts" in all fields relevant to the 2005 IHR (World Health Organization, 2008, pp. 14–15). They will be called upon to participate in an EC when necessary. Article 49 states that the DG shall select from the list of experts who will be part of the EC based on "their field of expertise and experience most relevant to the specific event that is taking place" (World Health Organization, 2008, pp. 31–32). On the basis of these mechanisms, international actions and guidelines are determined and will be transmitted and disseminated by networks of experts at the international and national level.

Experts During COVID-19: Identification of the Epistemic Community Network

SARS-CoV-2 virus causes the "severe acute respiratory syndrome coronavirus 2 (known as COVID-19)." Although new, it belongs to the coronavirus family identified by scientists in animals since the late 1930s. These include highly pathogenic viruses in livestock, laboratory animals, and pets (Drexler, Corman and Drosten, 2014). For a long time, coronaviruses were not considered harmful to humans. Scientific and medical experts recognised the danger posed by these viruses with the severe acute respiratory syndrome (SARS) outbreak in 2002/2003 (Drexler, Corman and Drosten, 2014; Fuk-Woo Chan, Kar-Pui Lau and Chiu-Yat Woo, 2013). After SARS, other human coronaviruses were detected: the HCoV-NL63 and HCoV-HKU1 in 2004 and 2005, and in 2012, MERS-CoV. The Middle East respiratory syndrome (MERS-CoV) caused the first coronavirus outbreak assessed under the 2005 IHR (Drexler, Corman and Drosten, 2014; Hilgenfeld and Peiris, 2013). MERS-CoV has been identified primarily in Middle Eastern countries, causing mild colds to more severe illnesses like SARS. However, some outbreaks have also shown a high mortality rate (Assiri, 2013; Lim, Lee and Rowe, 2013; WHO, 2013). Thus, although COVID-19 is new, it is part of a group of known viruses.

This antecedent is critical to recognising that before COVID-19 there were experts working on understanding these viruses. After the SARS outbreak, the WHO established the *Coronavirus Lab Network*, a group of 11 laboratories globally known as the first of its kind (World Health Organization, 2019). The network researched these pathogens, and part of its work was to develop a test for rapid virus identification (World Health Organization Multicentre Collaborative Network for Severe Acute Respiratory Syndrome (SARS)

Diagnosis, 2003). This network helped advance the global understanding of coronaviruses, establishing an epistemic community's foundation. Like other cases, the WHO has been a central actor in this epistemic community, acting as the group's coordinator. The coronavirus epistemic community members have been part of the WHO's body of expert advisors and have provided the organisation with information to confront other outbreaks.

When MERS-CoV emerged, people from this network participated in the core of the MERS-CoV epistemic community. Other groups in the epistemic community were: the Coronavirus Study Group (CSG) of the International Committee on Taxonomy of Viruses, which unified the scientific community and research by agreeing on the new pathogen's name (De Groot *et al.*, 2013); the WHO MERS-CoV Research Group (The WHO MERS-CoV Research Group, 2013); the MERS Emergency Committee established in July 2013; and the group of experts participating in WHO's technical consultations on MERS-CoV, WHO Blueprint Programme (World Health Organization, 2018).[3] The network, however, faced challenges, making it harder for it to consolidate its power to influence policymaking, and it did not strongly affect the international response. It could not position itself as a critical actor in the policymaking process (Coronado, 2019).

Even though the MERS-CoV outbreak signalled to the world the potential threat of these viruses, reaching fatality rates of 35% in 2019, the coronavirus epistemic community could not strengthen its influence within the WHO and other institutions. The problem was a lack of interest in researching SARS and similar viruses, along with problems to attract more funding (Condon and Patel, 2006).

The MERS-CoV epistemic community, as the predecessor of the current network in the context of the COVID-19 pandemic, provides the information to characterise the epistemic community for the latter (see Table 3.1).

Table 3.1 Characteristics of COVID-19 epistemic community

Common interest	Control COVID-19 transmission by implementing appropriate health and non-health measures based on evidence and understanding of the characteristics of the virus.
Epistemological belief	Given the high level of uncertainty, agreement on the urgency of the situation
Normative-principled beliefs	Reduce the number of deaths and severity of cases.
Causal beliefs	Find the best methods to identify the novel virus and the best interventions, including vaccines and potential treatments, to reduce the number of deaths and other costs associated with the pandemic.
Notions of validity	Shared norms, standards, and practices for identifying viruses and standardised methods to research and develop medical and non-medical interventions.

Source: Author's own elaboration

Therefore, the COVID-19 epistemic community included the WHO Emergency Committee COVID-19 created by the WHO (WHO, 2022) and groups such as the following:

- Advisory Group on Therapeutics Prioritization for COVID-19
- CSG of the International Committee on Taxonomy of Viruses
- COVID-19 IHR Emergency Committee
- COVID-19 Infection Prevention and Control Guidance Development Group
- GOARN
- Facilitation Council for the Access to COVID-19 Tools Accelerator
- Scientific Advisory Group on the Origins of Novel Pathogens
- Strategic Advisory Group of Experts on Immunization (SAGE)
- Technical Advisory Group (TAG) of Experts on Educational Institutions and COVID-19
- TAG on the COVID-19 Technology Access Pool
- TAG on COVID-19 Vaccine Composition
- Working Group on Ethics and COVID-19.

As a founding member of Pan-American Health Organization (PAHO) and the WHO and one of the WHO's 15 largest financial contributors (World Health Organization, 2020h), Mexico had access to the work done by these expert groups, and experts from the country had the channels to be part of them. Therefore, the Mexican government connects to the international epistemic community, and transgovernmental networks can disseminate global decisions and policies. These connections are through two main mechanisms. First, Mexican experts are part of expert lists created by the WHO due to their positions in the national bureaucracy, since the organisation requests some of these experts to be appointed by governments. This includes the IHR's National Focal Point (a technical area or person). Every six years, Mexico requests the addition of Mexican bureaucrats to the list of IHR experts; usually, these are officials working at the Ministry of Health. It should be noted that members on the IHR's list may or may not be called upon to collaborate with WHO.

Second, other experts outside Mexican public administration are invited directly by the WHO (Redaccion Aristegui Noticias, 2020; Villamil, 2020). In some cases, they must be endorsed by the Mexican government. Table 3.2 shows various Mexican experts appointed to some of these expert groups.

During COVID-19, Mexico had no direct representatives in the Emergency Committee. However, its main trading partners, the United States and Canada, did. The United States was represented by the Director of Migration and Quarantine of the Centres for Disease Control and Prevention (CDC), while Canada initially participated with the head of the Public

Table 3.2 Mexican experts participating in epistemic communities and trans-governmental networks connected to the WHO

Expert	Group	Year
Dr. Gerardo Varela	Member of the Influenza Centre Network	1952
Dr. José Ignacio Santos	Global Initiative on Sharing Avian Influenza Data (GISAID)	2010
Dr. Rogelio Pérez Padilla	H1N1 Influenza Emergency Committee	2009
Dr. Hugo López-Gatell	Response Review Committee to H1N1 Influenza	2011
Dr. Julio Frenk	WHO Interim Ebola Response Assessment Panel	2015
Dr. Ernesto Zedillo	Panel COVID-19	2020

Sources: Payne (1953); World Health Organization (2011a, 2011b, p. 77); World Health Organization-Panel of Independent Experts (July 2015); World Health Organization (2022)

Health Agency. Those countries provided direct access to Mexico's policy process at the global level. Over the years, the Mexican government has built a meaningful working relationship in health with its North American partners through transgovernmental networks. These include the North American Plan for Avian and Pandemic Influenza (Public Safety Canada, 2012) created after the SARS outbreak, the Global Health Security Initiative established after the 2001 bioterrorist attacks in the United States, and a network that has collaborated very closely with the WHO to develop policies for pandemic response.[4] These mechanisms connect the region to the global health process, facilitating policy transfer and information dissemination in decision-making.

Although it is not possible to name all the experts linked to these networks, it should be noted that on June 11, 2020, Mexico appointed Hugo López-Gatell, the Undersecretary of Prevention and Health Promotion, as the leader of the national response to COVID-19, who was also included in the list of experts of the 2005 IHR under Article 47 (Redaccion Animal Político, 2020). The Undersecretary has extensive experience in the field; he was involved in the response to the H1N1 pandemic influenza in 2009, contributing to the review process of the global response to the disease (see Table 3.1) and directly collaborating with North America's transgovernmental networks. Thus, he and other experts from the Health Secretariat were connected to the central global epistemic community.

In addition to this core group working within the federal government, the Mexican government convened a group of scientific advisors for COVID-19. Nonetheless, there is no clear information about who they were or how they were selected (Presidencia de la República Gobierno de México, 2020). Outside the national government, the third group of experts were primarily critics of the national strategy employed by the federal government, a group that emphasised the lack of compliance with international recommendations (Chertorivski *et al.*, 2020).

Therefore, Mexican experts are connected as members of a global epistemic community and a transgovernmental network, which, in theory, increases their ability to influence the adoption of global policies and recommendations at the national level. However, the next section will provide evidence that the Mexican response to COVID-19 did not always adhere to the guidelines proposed at the global level.

Mexico's Response to COVID-19

COVID-19 Epidemic in Mexico at a Glance

The COVID-19 epidemic in Mexico was initially long and challenging to control. The country faced structural problems with fragmented and unco-ordinated health systems and a lack of horizontality, while the government started an institutional reform based on an austerity policy and severe budget cuts for the health sector (Martinez and Nunez, 2021; Morales Fajardo and Cadena Inostroza, 2020; Orellana: 2020; Snake: 2020).

The complex epidemiological situation in the country contributed to the epidemic. In the early weeks of the pandemic, studies showed that the virus was more lethal in older adults and populations with comorbidities such as diabetes, obesity, and high blood pressure, characteristics present in Mexico's population (Aragón-Nogales, Vargas-Almanza and Miranda-Novales, 2019; Caldera-Villalobos *et al.*, 2020; Vargas-Vázquez *et al.*, 2021). These circumstances created a dramatic scene with more than 4.5 million cases and more than 300,000 deaths over 24 months (Johns Hopkins University, 2020), the fifth highest worldwide, with a mortality rate fluctuating between 10% and 60%.[5]

Early in 2021, Mexico obtained a relatively fast supply of vaccines due to its agreements with different pharmaceutical companies and governments, providing the country with a comprehensive portfolio of vaccines. Therefore, Mexico had a better situation early in the vaccine race than most countries in the Global South, leading to decreased cases after the vaccination roll-out. However, a slowdown in the supply of vaccines and the upsurge of new variants of concerns (VOCs), notably Delta and Omicron, created more waves and an upswing in cases. By mid-August 2021, cases reached levels previously seen during winter 2020–21 (one of the worst waves) (Figures 3.3 and 3.4) (Oxford University, 2020). With Omicron, in January 2022, case numbers saw new records, with more than 60,000 in one day (Oxford University, 2020; World Health Organization, 2020e).

Although this trend was similar worldwide, after more than 24 months of the epidemic, positivity rates (the number of positive cases relative to the number of tests done) were consistently high, reaching 60%, one of the highest in the world. Mexico remained one of the countries that applied the least tests, with an average of 35 per 1,000 per day (compared to similar countries, like Japan, with 77 per 1,000 per day) (Oxford University, 2020).

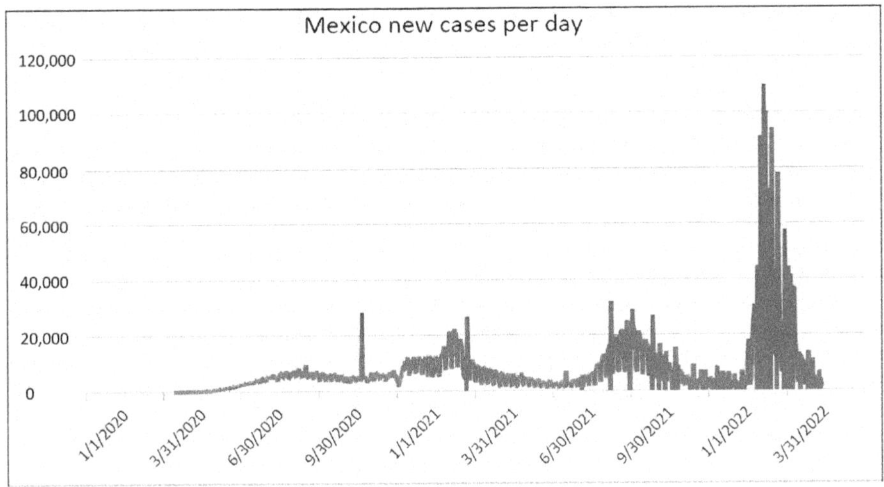

Figure 3.3 New cases per day with information from OurWorldinData.org (February 2020 to March 2022) (Oxford University, 2020)

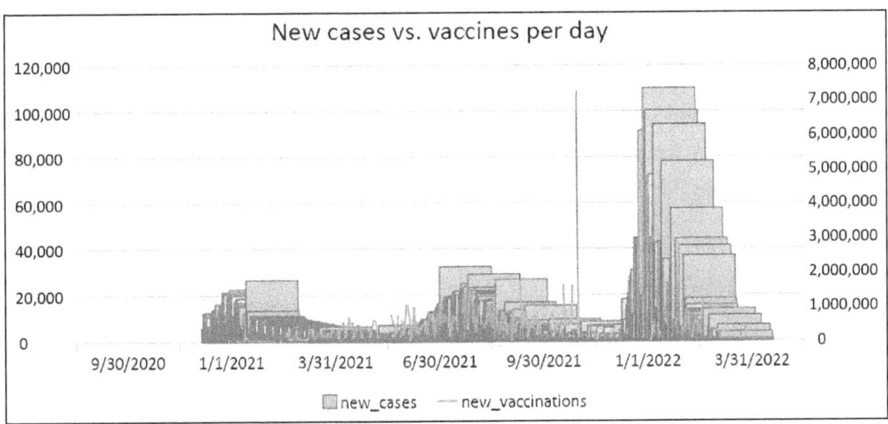

Figure 3.4 Daily COVID-19 vaccine doses per day and new cases in Mexico (Oxford University, 2020)

Government Response

On December 31, 2019, China officially notified the WHO of atypical pneumonia in Wuhan (Han *et al.*, 2020; Lopez-Ortiz, 2020). Due to the evolution of the situation and following the 2005 IHR, the organisation called an Emergency Committee (EC). On January 30, 2020, after the Second EC Meeting, the WHO's DG declared the COVID-19 outbreak a PHEIC (World Health Organization, 2020f). On March 11, after weeks of sustained transmission and the emergence of more epidemics in different parts of the world (World Health

Organization, 2020f), the WHO concluded that the COVID-19 outbreak had reached pandemic status (World Health Organization, 2020b, 2020d).

Unlike the H1N1 influenza pandemic in 2009, when Mexico was the first to notify cases internationally, placing the country at the centre of the pandemic and the international response, Mexico did not have a predominant position during COVID-19. Whereas the H1N1 pandemic forced a decision-making process where all levels of government worked together throughout the epidemic, the situation with COVID-19 did not trigger the same level of domestic collaboration.

The government's initial response was cautiously preventive rather than aggressive. The first official meeting to discuss the outbreak was held on January 30 with the National Committee for Health Security and the WHO's International Adviser on Health Emergencies (Secretaria de Salud Mexico, 2020). The first case was detected in the country on February 27 (BBC News Mundo, 2020), and two more related cases were confirmed the following day. All these identified patients attended the same conference in Bergamo, Italy (BBC News Mundo, 2020), the country that was the pandemic's epicentre during the first wave. Meanwhile, the Mexican government asked the population to be calmed, affirming that COVID-19 was a mild disease (BBC News Mundo, 2020).

Only after the WHO declared a pandemic on March 18, 2020, did the legal and extended cabinet members meet with the National Committees for Emergencies and Health Security, chaired by the Secretary of Safety and Citizen Protection and the Secretary of Health (Álvarez, 2020). The official response was announced the following day when the General Health Council (GHC)[6] issued a decree recognising the epidemic in Mexico and publishing the response mechanisms to manage it (Diario Contra Réplica, 2020). Under this decree, the federal Secretary of Health assumed the national leadership, and on March 30, it presented to the GHC a package of health security measures to face the pandemic. The document also emphasised that the country's actions would be based on information provided by WHO and international experts (Secretaria de Gobernación México, 2020).

The GHC's role was active at the beginning of the pandemic, issuing a series of decrees published in the Official Journal of the Federation (Diario Oficial de la Federación). These included the following[7]:

- March 23, 2020, Recognition of COVID-19 as a disease of national concern
- March 30, 2020, Declaration of a national health emergency due to COVID-19
- March 31, 2020, Issuance of extraordinary measures to combat COVID-19
- May 14, 2020, Establishment of a strategy for reopening the economy and a four-tier colour-coded COVID-19 risk assessment scale

The GHC mainly addressed issues related to the functioning of the government early in the epidemic, and there is no clear evidence that it played a more prominent role in the subsequent months.

The Role of Epistemic Communities in the Adoption of Global Measures during the Response to COVID-19 in Mexico

According to studies on epistemic communities and transgovernmental networks, the presence of members of expert networks in a national government increases the likelihood of adopting and complying with policies and guidelines derived from global governance during a crisis such as the COVID-19 pandemic. When the virus emerged, Mexico was connected to these networks. Therefore, disseminating global policies to respond to COVID-19 was expected to reach a high level of decision-making, increasing their adoption and implementation at the national level. Many of those connected to transgovernmental networks and epistemic communities were also directly involved in the government, playing a dual position as experts and bureaucrats. For instance, the Undersecretary of Prevention and Health Promotion was appointed as the head of the national response. He used his expert position to legitimise political decisions without prioritising global economic and public health policy recommendations (Culebro, 2020, p. 50).

At the same time, other expert voices emerged at the national level, questioning the government's strategy. Among these experts, five former Secretaries of Health, including former secretary Julio Frenk, an academic with an international reputation and highly connected to the global epistemic community, joined a group of renowned specialists as an opposition group (Chertorivski *et al.*, 2020).

There was a belief before the COVID-19 pandemic that the legitimacy of scientific knowledge usually makes it widely accepted by society; however, the theory of epistemic community recognises that science can be politically motivated (Clark and Majone, 1985). In Mexico, a country amid political change, the president's views dominated the decision-making process during the pandemic, even though the Mexican laws had created the figure of the GHC for a health emergency as a more impartial and expert-guided decision-making instrument. Thus, at the beginning of the pandemic, the GHC endorsed experts to oversee emergency management and make recommendations based on their scientific knowledge. However, the president set the tone and determined which actions were to be followed or not by the country. For instance, he decided to implement an early economic reopening, ignoring guidelines published on May 12, 2020, by the WHO, which established that an epidemic was controlled when a positivity rate (the number of positive cases in relation to the number of tests done) reached below 5% (World Health Organization, 2020c). In Mexico, however, the end of the National Day of *Sana Distancia* on May 30, 2020, meant a gradual economic reopening of the formal sector—since social distancing was not imposed at the individual level (Anda-Jauregui, 2020). At the same time, positivity rates fluctuated between 40% and 60%, with just a few brief moments flattening the cases' curve (Oxford University, 2020). Many blamed the president for not allowing stricter confinement measures to be established and for making constant statements minimising the pandemic since the beginning (AFP

Ciudad de Mexico, 2020). In February 2020, he declared that Mexicans should continue to visit restaurants, contrary to international guidelines (Burki, 2020).

The experts working for the government and critical actors connected to the national epistemic community with the international one had implicitly accepted the president's actions over global recommendations, as the following analysis of specific policies will illustrate.

Testing

Testing has been one of the key measures to control the pandemic. The WHO stated, "Diagnostic testing for SARS-CoV-2 is a critical component to the overall prevention and control strategy for COVID-19 (World Health Organization, 2021a)." Together with contact tracing and isolation of cases, this strategy has been crucial to breaking transmission chains (World Health Organization, 2021b). Testing became an essential component of the international measures recommended by the WHO. On March 16, 2020, the WHO's DG mentioned during a briefing the phrase "test, test, test" as a necessary strategy to deal with the pandemic and to control the spread of the virus, pointing out to countries with more widespread outbreaks of the need to carry out more tests (World Health Organization, 2020c). In addition, experts started publishing about the importance of testing for controlling the epidemic (Araz *et al.*, 2020; Mercer and Salit, 2021; Rosenthal, 2020), reinforcing the WHO's guidance with scientific evidence.

Nonetheless, there were limited capacities worldwide to detect the virus at the beginning of the pandemic. In June 2020, the WHO established the WHO COVID-19 Reference Laboratory Network to support testing capacities worldwide, track changes in the virus, and develop new methods, assays, and testing protocols (World Health Organization, 2020f). One of the laboratories participating in the network was Mexico's Institute of Diagnosis and Epidemiological Reference (Instituto de Diagnóstico y Referencia Epidemiológicos–InDRE), part of the Federal Secretariat of Health (World Health Organization, 2020f).

Even though Mexico participates in the network, the federal government decided to apply a limited number of tests for COVID-19, a trend that continued during the pandemic. In August 2020, Mexico ranked 150th globally with 8,500 tests per 1,000,000 inhabitants; by January 2022, the country had fallen to 166th with 104,417 tests per 1,000,000 (Worldometer, 2022). Moreover, contact tracing over time was limited in the country (Hale *et al.*, 2021, p. 1; Oxford University, 2020).

The topic was controversial since the expert leader of the response in Mexico declared that doing more tests "would be a waste of time, effort and resources and is a distraction from surveillance, prevention and control efforts (Milenio,

2020; Robles de la Rosa, 2020)," a posture that at first seemed to be supported by the WHO/PAHO representative in Mexico (United Nations Information Centre, 2020). The WHO took a cautious approach, considering that testing capacities were limited worldwide (World Health Organization, 2020a, 2020d). Whereas in March 2020, lab capacity and availability of tests were recognised as challenges for implementing broader testing strategies, the organisation emphasised the importance of understanding each country's situation and defining public health interventions (World Health Organization, 2020g).

In this sense, in July 2020, the WHO's International Advisor on Health Emergencies, Jean-Marc Gabastou, recommended that Mexico's government increase its diagnostic capacity and test application (Chavez, 2020). Gabastou requested that authorities make "all possible efforts" to save lives, noting that "the high exposure of the Mexican population to comorbid factors . . . places the country in a very high level of vulnerability" (Chavez, 2020). The expert in health emergencies warned that, although the measures that the government of Mexico and its health authorities took on time allowed the health system to remain "resilient," they needed to improve various aspects because the most complex thing was coming. It was not until August 24 that the government modified the definition of cases to increase the number of tests (Vergara, 2020).

Many questioned the Mexican government's lack of testing. The expert in charge of pandemic management—the Undersecretary of Prevention and Health Promotion—insisted that the number of tests done in Mexico was adequate to assess the epidemic. He also clarified that the policy was not due to a lack of resources or budget cuts. In an interview on May 4, he added that "the tests have one objective: epidemiological surveillance . . . if severe cases are recorded at 100%, then 100% must be tested. So (he wondered) is there a limit on the number of tests? How many severe cases are there?" he noted (Latinus, 2020; Robles de la Rosa, 2020; United Nations Information Centre, 2020). His position was contrary to the recommendations of many public health experts.

Use of Face Masks

The use of face masks among the population was initially controversial because of the fear of driving excess demand that could cause a shortage in the health sector. Further research on the topic (and production increases) led to a change in this measure. The WHO recommended the general use of face masks on June 5, 2020, based on scientific evidence showing (CDC, 2020) its advantages for the entire population. However, face masks were not widely recommended in Mexico until very late in the pandemic (Chen Keung, Hing Lam and Leung, 2020; World Health Organization, 2020a). For the leader at the federal level, this type of protective equipment provided a false sense of security and insisted that other measures, such as social distancing from other people and constantly washing hands, were more critical. The decision also came amid the controversy of July 24, 2020, when the president declared that he was not wearing face masks because their efficacy was not scientifically proven. He pointed out that national experts responsible for managing the pandemic in Mexico did not recommend it to him. Finally, in November 2020 (Pavon, 2020; Redaccion Animal Político, 2020), the importance of face masks was acknowledged, but only on a voluntary basis, not as a compulsory norm like in other countries. The justification of this decision was based on accounts of the abuse of authority of previous governments (Perusquia, 2020; Navarro, 2020), an argument consistent with the political ideology of the current government and unrelated to scientific evidence or international guidance (Perusquia, 2020).

In this context, other measures represented a significant challenge for the Mexican population, such as the country's clean water shortage and the importance of the informal sector in the economy. While a water problem was recognised at the beginning of the pandemic, the federal Undersecretary of Health assigned the responsibility only to states and municipalities, even though the WHO and other international organisations have expressed that guaranteeing access to this resource was of the utmost importance to fight epidemics. Again, the political argument outweighed the technical recommendation and evidence-based solutions. As for the "healthy distance" and staying at home, it should be noted that most of the infections occurred in highly populated areas, where informal trade abounds, with low wages, making people less willing to stay at home, making social distancing more difficult (Chang, Hong and Varley, 2020; Otto *et al.*, 2020). These factors strongly called into question the reasons behind not enforcing face masks, given the existence of scientific evidence and the international epistemic community's acceptance. However, the use of face masks was common among the population in Mexico, mainly because state and local governments established mandates or recommendations.

The Burden of the Pandemic on Children

The impact of the pandemic on children has been continuously analysed since this sector of the population initially seemed to be less exposed to the disease, and there were fewer cases with catastrophic outcomes. Nonetheless, during the evolution of the pandemic, more children were affected by the disease, and, whether symptomatic or asymptomatic, they could increase transmissibility in some settings (e.g., households with extended families). In Mexico, however, children were not considered a vulnerable population. Therefore, they were not targeted in the national strategy. This decision created controversy and questioned the actions of national experts working with the government in implementing specific policies, such as the government's plan for returning to school at the end of August 2021. Whereas multiple arguments support the reopening of schools at the international level, many questioned if Mexico had the conditions for a "safe return to school." Even when cases were rising among children in different parts of the world due to new VOCs, such as the *Delta* variant (Borter, 2021), the Secretary of Health published in different social media outlets an advertisement affirming that "In the world, there is no evidence of a COVID-19 epidemic among children" (Gobierno de México, 2021) (see Figure 3.5). At the same time, the president and federal leader declared that there was not enough evidence that children should be vaccinated (Carrillo, 2021).

With the rise of the new VOC *Omicron*, children became the target of multiple vaccination campaigns worldwide, rushing governments to verify and approve vaccines for children under 18. The transmissibility levels of Omicron increased the number of cases in winter 2022. Although the variant seemed less aggressive than Delta, it spread faster, causing millions of

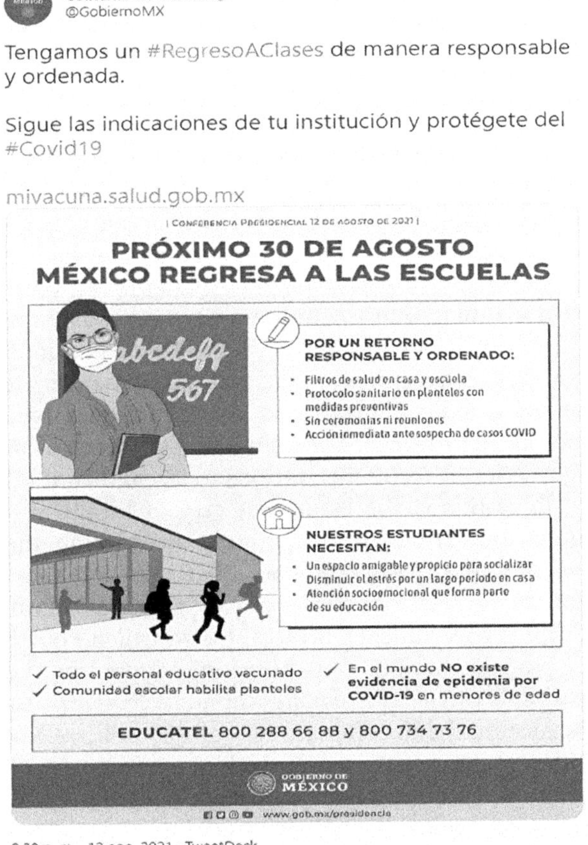

Figure 3.5 Government of Mexico Publication on Twitter about the Pandemic and Children (Gobierno de México @GobiernoMX, 2021)

cases in a few weeks, including thousands of cases among children. Under these circumstances, the expert leading the response in Mexico insisted children were at a lower risk of dying due to COVID-19 and, at the same time, affirmed that the WHO did not recommend vaccination for children (Lopez-Gatell, 2020). However, his interpretation of WHO's recommendations published on his official Facebook page in December 2021 was misleading and erroneous since the WHO recognised the importance of vaccination in children to reduce transmission and protect vulnerable sectors. The WHO, however, was trying to address the lack of available vaccines in developing countries by convincing countries to send over supplies of vaccines to these countries by not overemphasising vaccination in children. Therefore, the Mexican expert connected to the international epistemic community network and, with the capacity to influence the adoption of global recommendations, interpreted them according to the national political strategy, which was inconsistent with the scientific evidence or international advice.

Effects of Politics on the Epistemic Community Network

The actions previously described created a divisive atmosphere in the national epistemic community network. The government amplified national divisions by not accepting criticism or refusing to enter a dialogue with national experts with different ideas, despite being recognised experts in their field and being directly connected to the transgovernmental network. At the same time, the government kept claiming that the national strategy was based on scientific evidence and in compliance with the WHO's recommendations. Government experts were severely questioned for the lack of consistency with the measures recommended globally. This caused several national experts to express their concern about the strategy, criticising the management of the epidemic and presenting a series of recommendations to strengthen it (Castellano Ballestero, 2020). In response, the Undersecretary of Health discredited these recommendations and criticised this group, questioning their experience as public servants and experts (Infobae, 2020) and feeding the discourse that every critic of the national strategy had specific political interests and opposed the current government's project, the so-called Fourth Transformation (Aristegui Noticias, 2020). This position, adopted by the government, weakened the ability of the epistemic community network to have a more significant influence on the dissemination of global policies.

Similarly, other experts criticised the lack of evidence, lack of data, disorganised information, and disparities between the figures presented between states and the federation; this last issue raised questions about the accuracy in the number of cases (Agren, 2020; Aristegui Noticias, 2020; Daen, 2020; Weiss, 2020). Given the different perspectives, it is possible to assert that opposed or rival expert groups to the government's own experts emerged and provided a different interpretation of the WHO's recommendations. In the absence of consensus among the national epistemic community, the legitimacy of the government's experts was affected. The population received conflicting messages, leading them to follow those measures that suited their personal interests and that were sustainable with their available resources.

Finally, another critical aspect of the politicisation of pandemic management in Mexico was daily conferences to communicate information on the response to the epidemic in the country, which served to legitimise the current government through the pandemic response officer and experts from the epistemic community. These conferences were not solely for presenting the technical response but used to promote actions implemented to confront the pandemic as political successes (Llano Guibarra and Águila Sánchez, 2020). A prominent case in point was the presidential announcement of the appointment of the Undersecretary of Health Promotion to the IHR's list of experts. This was an unprecedented action, given that other experts who had been previously appointed to this list never received such political visibility. At the same time, the appointment of another expert from the National Institute of Public Health as a member of the Expert Group on Strategic Advice (SAGE) on COVID-19 vaccines from June 2020 to December 2021 was never even mentioned at this level (INSP, 2020).[8] Both appointments were equally important and should have been presented as achievements of the network of national experts; however, how the information was officially treated mainly favoured the image of the national expert in charge of leading the federal pandemic response strategy.

The dual role of experts working for the Mexican government led to conflicts of interest within the community and contradictions that hindered an appropriate response to COVID-19. It also limited the capacity to disseminate and transfer global policies to manage the pandemic. Even though international guidelines were continuously evolving and adapting to the most updated scientific evidence, it did not seem necessary that this should be the same in the case of Mexico.

Conclusion

The examples above highlight epistemic communities' problems in disseminating and transferring global policies. In global health governance, epistemic communities and transgovernmental networks are important mechanisms that help transfer and disseminate policies created at the global level. Their connections facilitate the dissemination of standards and the transmission of information. Although expert networks can influence public policy at all levels, factors in their internal structure and the way they connect to the decision-making process can limit this ability. In the case of Mexico, we confirm that the national actors linked to the transnational networks of experts faced problems due to the lack of cohesion and consensus, but mostly to political interference, which affected their legitimacy. This work reaffirms a fine line between power and knowledge and that expert groups can use their role as authorities on an issue to promote a political ideology even if it does not resonate with science. Although the Mexican government adopted various international recommendations, it also decided to place less emphasis on proven measures, such as the use of face masks, mandatory confinement, and total closure of economic activity.

In this case (as in other countries), global policies derived from evidence-based recommendations were scrutinised and discredited. Furthermore, the government imposed a decision-making model based on national-state interests even when facing phenomena requiring a coordinated global response and coordination with other state and non-state actors, which is indispensable to facing pandemics. There was a clear domination of symbolic politics supported by a narrative that has been governing the policymaking process in Mexico, where presidentialism is probably stronger than ever.

The analysis of the experience with COVID-19 in various contexts will allow us to reassess the functioning of epistemic communities and transgovernmental networks as providers of scientific evidence in decision-making. It will also be necessary to test whether the dual role of expert and decision-maker is essential for decision-making effectiveness or is more important to promote mechanisms where experts connect to governments only through global actors and somehow can be isolated from national politics, such as expert groups affiliated to international organisations.

Notes

1 This chapter is a continuation of the work published as Coronado Martínez (2021).
2 In addition, for the first time, it includes the possibility for other non-state actors or individuals to report to WHO on the likely occurrence of cases of a disease with pandemic potential or a new disease. See Article 9 of the International Health Regulations.
3 Given the complexity of networks, this research only identifies those that were central, and it acknowledges that there may have been others involved.
4 See Epidemic Intelligence from Open Sources EIOS. Available at: www.who.int/initiatives/eios (Accessed January 20, 2021).
5 Data from January 2022.
6 Consejo de Salud General—GSC in Spanish.
7 The agreements can be found at https://dof.gob.mx/.
8 An updated list of the members is www.who.int/groups/strategic-advisory-group-of-experts-on-immunization/working-groups/covid-19.

References

Adler, E. and Haas, P. (1992) 'Epistemic communities, world-order, and the creation of a reflective research program conclusion', *International Organization*, 46(1), pp. 367–390.

AFP Ciudad de Mexico (2020) 'Los pecados originales que prolongan la pandemia en México', *La Prensa*, 23 July. [Online]. Available at: www.prensa.com/mundo/los-pecados-originales-que-prolongan-la-pandemia-en-mexico/ (Accessed 25 August 2020).

Agren, D. (2020) 'Mexico flying blind as lack of COVID-19 testing mystifies experts', *The Guardian*, 24 July. [Online]. Available at: www.theguardian.com/global-development/2020/jul/24/mexico-covid-19-testing-coronavirus (Accessed 2 September 2020).

Alexander, G. & Bennett, A. (2005) *Case studies and theory development in social sciences*. Cambridge: MIT Press.

Álvarez, E. (2020) 'Se reúnen comités nacionales de Emergencia y Seguridad en Salud por Covid-19', *MVS Noticias*, 19 March. [Online]. Available at: https://mvsnoticias.com/nacional/2020/3/19/se-reunen-comites-nacionales-de-emergencia-seguridad-en-salud-por-covid-19-434808.html (Accessed 10 September 2020).

Anda-Jauregui, G.D. (2020) COVID-19 in Mexico: a network of epidemics. *Física y Sociedad*, p. 2.

Antoniades, A. (2003) 'Epistemic communities, epistemes and the construction of world politics', *Global Society*, 1(17), pp. 21–38.

Aragón-Nogales, R., Vargas-Almanza, I. and Miranda-Novales, M.G. (2019) 'COVID-19 por SARS-CoV-2: la nueva emergencia de salud', *Revista Mexicana de Pediatría*, 86(6), pp. 213–218.

Araz, O. *et al.* (2020) 'The importance of widespread testing for COVID-19 pandemic: systems thinking for drive-through testing sites', *Health Systems*, 9(2), pp. 119–123.

Aristegui Noticias (2020) 'Critica AMLO a quienes "se vuelven expertos", desinforman y mienten sobre coronavirus', *Aristegui Noticias*, 13 March. [Online]. Available at: https://aristeguinoticias.com/1303/mexico/critica-amlo-a-quienes-desinforman-se-vuelven-expertos-y-mienten-sobre-coronavirus/ (Accessed 30 August 2020).

Assiri, A.A. (2013) 'Epidemiological, demographic, and clinical characteristics of 47 cases of middle east respiratory syndrome coronavirus disease from Saudi Arabia: a descriptive study', *The Lancet*, 13, pp. 752–760.

BBC News Mundo (2020) 'Coronavirus en México: confirman los primeros casos de COVID-19 en el país', *BBC News Mundo*, 29 February. [Online]. Available at: www.bbc.com/mundo/noticias-america-latina-51677751#:~:text=M%C3%A9xico%20confirm%C3%B3%20el%20viernes%20sus,que%20recientemente%20estuvo%20en%20Italia (Accessed 29 August 2020).

Behrmann, S. and Santucci, J. (2020) 'Here's a timeline of President Donald Trump's and Dr. Anthony Fauci's relationship', *USA Today*, 28 October. [Online]. Available at: www.usatoday.com/story/news/politics/2020/10/28/president-donald-trump-anthony-fauci-timeline-relationship-coronavirus-pandemic/3718797001/ (Accessed 25 November 2020).

Berry, F.S. and Berry, W.D. (2007) 'Innovation and diffusion models', in Sabatier, P. (ed.) *Policy research in theories of the policy process*. 2nd edn. New York: Routledge, pp. 219–257.

Borter, G. (2021) 'Children hospitalized with COVID-19 hits record number in U.S. amid Delta variant surge', *Reuters*, 16 August. [Online]. Available at: www.reuters.com/world/us/children-hospitalized-with-covid-19-us-hits-record-number-2021-08-14/#:~:text=Aug%2014%20(Reuters)%20%2D%20The,the%20highly%20transmissible%20Delta%20variant (Accessed 30 August 2021).

Burki, T. (2020) 'COVID-19 in Latin America', *The Lancet*, 20(5), pp. 547–548.

Caldera-Villalobos, C. *et al.* (2020) 'The coronavirus disease (COVID-19) challenge in Mexico: a critical and forced reflection as individuals and society', *Public Health*, 8(333).

Carrillo, E. (2021) 'Sin evidencia que niños necesiten vacuna contra COVID-19, afirma SSA', *Forbes Mexico*, 27 July. [Online]. Available at: www.forbes.com.mx/sin-evidencia-que-ninos-necesiten-vacuna-contra-covid-19-afirma-salud/ (Accessed 31 August 2021).

Castellano Ballestero, A. (2020) 'Ex secretarios de Salud advierten que actuación de gobierno ante COVID-19 es confusa', *MVS Noticias*, 7 May. [Online]. Available at: https://mvsnoticias.com/nacional/2020/5/7/ex-secretarios-de-salud-advierten-que-actuacion-de-gobierno-ante-covid-19-es-confusa-439396.html (Accessed 30 August 2020).

CDC (2020) 'CDC COVID-19'. Available at: www.cdc.gov/coronavirus/2019-ncov/index.html (Accessed 30 August 2020).

Chang, R., Hong, J. and Varley, K. (2020) 'The COVID resilience ranking', *Bloomberg*, 21 December. [Online]. Available at: www.bloomberg.com/graphics/covid-resilience-ranking/#xj4y7vzkg (Accessed 21 December 2020).

Chavez, V. (2020) 'OMS y OPS alertan: "en México, lo peor del COVID está por llegar"', *El Financiero*, 11 June. [Online]. Available at: www.elfinanciero.com.mx/nacional/oms-y-ops-alertan-en-mexico-lo-peor-del-covid-esta-por-llegar/ (Accessed 29 August 2020).

Chen Keung, K., Hing Lam, T. and Leung, C.C.L. (2020) 'Wearing face masks in the community during the COVID-19 pandemic: altruism and solidarity', *The Lancet*, 399. [Online]. Available at: www.thelancet.com/pdfs/journals/lancet/PIIS0140-6736(20)30918-1.pdf.

Chertorivski, S. *et al.* (2020) *La gestión de la pandemia en México: análisis preliminar y recomendaciones urgentes.* Mexico City: Consejo Consultivo Ciudadano Pensando en México.

Clark, W. and Majone, G. (1985) 'The critical appraisal of scientific inquiries with policy implications', *Science, Technology and Human Values*, 10(3), pp. 6–19.

Condon, R. and Patel, M. (2006) 'Response of the western pacific regional office', in *SARS how a global epidemic was stopped.* Geneva: World Health Organization Western Pacific Region, pp. 49–55.

Conly, J. *et al.* (2020) 'Use of medical face masks versus particulate respirators as a component of personal protective equipment for health care workers in the context of the COVID-19 pandemic', *Antimicrobial Resistance and Infection Control*, 9(126), pp. 1–7. Available at: https://link.springer.com/content/pdf/10.1186/s13756-020-00779-6.pdf.

Coronado, M.E. (2019) *The international response to disease outbreaks: the relevance of epistemic communities in international cooperation.* Ottawa: Carleton University.

Coronado, M.E. (2021) 'La gobernanza global de la salud y los límites de las redes de expertos en la respuesta al brote de la Covid-19 Mexico', *Foro Internacional*, LXI(2), pp. 469–505.

Cozzens, S. and Woodhouse, E. (1995) 'Science, government, and the politics of knowledge', in Jasanoff, S. (ed.) *Handbook of science and technology studies.* Thousand Oaks: Sage, pp. 532–553.

Culebro, J.E. (2020) 'Gestión de crisis y retos para el sistema de salud. La coordinación vertical y horizontal para los sistemas de salud en México', *Reporte CESOP*, 132, pp. 44–52.

Daen, A. (2020) 'Los vigilantes: expertos en datos evalúan la forma en que salud ha informado sobre covid-19 en México', *Animal político*, 5 May. [Online]. Available at: https://www.animalpolitico.com/2020/05/salud-datos-pandemia-expertos-covid-coronavirus/ (Accessed 10 September 2020).

Davis Cross, M.K. (2013) 'Rethinking epistemic communities twenty years later', *Review of International Studies*, I(39), pp. 137–160.

De Groot, R.J. *et al.* (2013, July) 'Middle east respiratory syndrome coronavirus (MERS-CoV): announcement of the coronavirus study group', *Journal of Virology*, 87(14), pp. 7790–7792.

Deacon, B. (2007) 'The social policy of international non-state actors', in Deacon, B. (ed.) *Global social policy & government*. Los Angeles: Sage, pp. 88–108.

Diario Contra Réplica (2020) 'Primera reunión del Consejo de Salubridad General por coronavirus', *Diario Contra Replica*, 19 March. [Online]. Available at: www.contrareplica.mx/nota-Primera-reunion-del-Consejo-de-Salubridad-General-por-coronavirus202019355 (Accessed 30 August 2020).

Dodgson, R. and Lee, K. (2002) 'Global health governance: a conceptual review', in *Global governance. Critical perspectives*. New York: Routledge, pp. 92–110.

Dolowitz, D. and Marsh, D. (1996) 'Who learns what from whom? A review of the policy transfer literature', *Political Studies*, XLIV, pp. 343–357.

Drexler, J.F., Corman, V.M. and Drosten, C. (2014) 'Ecology, evolution and classification of bat coronaviruses in the aftermath of SARS', *Antiviral Research*, 101, pp. 45–56.

Dunlop, C. (2009) 'Policy transfer as learning: capturing variation in what decision-makers learn from epistemic communities', *Policy Studies*, 30(3), pp. 289–311.

Evans, M. (2004) 'Understanding policy transfer', in Evans, M. (ed.) *Policy transfer in global perspective*. Aldershot: Ashgate, pp. 10–42.

Fidler, D.P. (2010) *The challenges of global health governance*. New York: Council on Foreign Relations, pp. 3–10.

Fleming, N. (2020) 'Coronavirus misinformation, and how scientists can help to fight it', *Nature*, 17 June.

Frenk, J. and Moon, S. (2013) 'Governance challenges in global health', *New England Journal of Medicine*, 368(10), pp. 936–942.

Fuk-Woo Chan, J., Kar-Pui Lau, S. and Chiu-Yat Woo, P. (2013) 'The emerging novel middle east respiratory syndrome coronavirus: the "knowns" and "unknowns", *Journal of the Formosan Medical Association*, 112, pp. 372–381.

Gobierno de México (2021) 'Pandemia sí afecta a menores de edad, es falso lo que dice el gobierno—publicidad'. [Online]. Available at: www.animalpolitico.com/elsabueso/menores-pandemia-covid-infografia-gobierno-falso/ (Accessed 30 August 2021).

Gobierno de México (@GobiernoMX) (2021) 'Tengamos un #RegresoAClases de manera responsable y ordenada. Sigue las indicaciones de tu institución y protégete del #Covid19 mivacuna.salud.gob.mx', *Twitter*, 12 agosto, 9:30 pm.

Haas, P. (1992) 'Introduction: epistemic communities and international policy coordination', *International Organization*, 46(1), pp. 1–35.

Haas, P. (2004, August) 'When does power listen to the truth? A constructivist approach to the policy process', *Journal of European Public Policy*, 11(4), pp. 569–592.

Haas, P. (2015) *Epistemic communities, constructivism, and international environmental politics*. 1st edn. New York: Routledge.

Hale, T. *et al.* (2021) 'A global panel database of pandemic policies (Oxford COVID-19 government response tracker)', *Nature Human Behaviour*.

Hallal, P.C. (2021) 'SOS Brazil: science under attack', *The Lancet*, 397(10272), pp. 373–374.

Han, W. *et al.* (2020) 'The course of clinical diagnosis and treatment of a case infected with coronavirus disease 2019', *Journal of Medical Virology*, 92(5), pp. 461–463.

Hasenclever, A.E.A. (2000) 'Integrating theories of international regimes', *Review of International Studies*, 26, pp. 3–33.

Hilgenfeld, R. and Peiris, M. (2013) 'From SARS to MERS: 10 years of research on highly pathogenic human coronaviruses', *Antiviral Research*, 100, pp. 286–295.

Horton, R. (2020) 'Offline: science and politics in the era of COVID-19', *The Lancet*, 396(10259), p. 1319.

Infobae (2020) 'López-Gatell arremetió contra ex secretarios de Salud: nunca se familiarizaron con la vigilancia epidemiológica', *Infobae*, 24 September. [Online]. Available at: www.infobae.com/america/mexico/2020/09/24/lopez-gatell-arremetio-contra-ex-secretarios-de-salud-que-criticaron-la-estrategia-covid-nunca-se-familiarizaron-con-la-vigilancia-epidemiologica/ (Accessed 15 March 2021).

INSP (Instituto Nacional de Salud Publica) (2020) *La Dra. Celia Alpuche se integra al Grupo de Expertos en Asesoramiento Estratégico de la OMS*, July 10. Mexico City. Available at: https://www.insp.mx/avisos/5434-grupo-expertos-asesoramiento-estrategico-oms.html

Jenson, J. (2010) 'Diffusing ideas after neoliberalism: the social investment perspective in Europe and Latin America', *Global Social Policy*, 10(1), pp. 59–84.

Johns Hopkins University (2020) 'COVID-19 map Johns Hopkins coronavirus resource center'. [Online]. Available at: https://coronavirus.jhu.edu/map.html (Accessed 15 September 2021).

Kamradt-Scott, A. (2013) 'The politics of medicine and the global governance of pandemic influenza', *International Journal of Health Services*, 43(1), pp. 105–121.

Karlsson, M. (2004) 'Epistemic communities and cooperative security: the case of communicable disease control in the Baltic Sea region', *Journal of International and Area Studies*, 11(1), pp. 79–100.

Keck, M. and Sikkink, K. (1999) 'Transnational advocacy networks in international and regional politics', *International Social Science Journal*, 159, pp. 89–101.

Keohane, R.O. and Nye, J.S. (1974) 'Transgovernmental relations and international organizations', *World Politics*, 27(1), pp. 39–62.

Kurowska, X. and Kratochwill, F. (2012) 'The social constructivism sensibility and CSDP research', in Kurowska, X. and Breuer, F. (eds.) *Explaining the EU's common security and defence policy. Theory in action*. London: Palgrave MacMillan.

Latinus (2020) 'López-Gatell explica por qué en México no se hacen más pruebas de COVID-19', *Latinus*, 14 May. [Online]. Available at: https://latinus.us/2020/05/14/lopez-gatell-explica-mexico-no-hacen-mas-pruebas-covid/ (Accessed 15 August 2020).

Lee, L. and Fidler, D. (2007) 'Avian and pandemic influenza: progress and problems with global health governance', *Global Public Health*, 2(3), pp. 215–234.

Legrand, T. (2015) 'Transgovernmental policy networks in the anglosphere', *Public Administration*, 93(4), pp. 973–991.

Legrand, T. (2019) 'Sovereignty renewed: transgovernmental policy networks and the global local dilemma', in Stone, D.S. and Moloney, K. (eds.) *Global policy and transnational administration*. Oxford: Oxford University Press, pp. 200–222.

Lennox, V. (2008) *Conceptualising global governance in international relations*. Ottawa: E-International Relations.

Lewis, D. (2022) 'Why did the WHO take two years to say COVID is airborne', *Nature*, 604, pp. 26–31. [Online]. Available at: www.nature.com/articles/d41586-022-00925-7#:~:text=These%20droplets%20contaminate%20nearby%20surfaces,and%20linger%20in%20the%20air (Accessed 15 August 2020).

Lim, L.P., Lee, T.H. and Rowe, E.K. (2013) 'Middle east respiratory syndrome coronavirus (MERS CoV): update 2013', *Current Infectious Disease Reports*, 15, pp. 295–298.

Llano Guibarra, N.I. and Águila Sánchez, J.C. (2020) 'Conferencias de prensa y COVID-19: exploring the Mexican government response from health communication', *Revista Española de Comunicación en Salud*, 1, p. 138.

Löblová, O. (2018) 'When epistemic communities fail: exploring the mechanism of policy influence', *Policy Studies Journal*, 46(1), pp. 160–189.

Lopez-Gatell, H. (2020) 'Facebook personal page'. [Online]. (Accessed 15 January 2022).

Lopez-Ortiz, E. (2020) 'From the handling of an outbreak by an unknown pathogen in Wuhan to the preparedness and response in the face of the emergence of COVID-19 in Mexico', *Gaceta Médica de México*, 156(2), pp. 132–137.

Majone, G. (1989) *Evidence, argument, and persuasion in the policy process.* New Haven: Yale University Press.

Mandavilli, A. (2020) 'WHO to review evidence of airborne transmission of coronavirus', *The New York Times*, 6 July. [Online]. Available at: www.nytimes.com/2020/07/07/health/coronavirus-aerosols-who.html (Accessed 30 August 2020).

Martinez, J. and Nunez, L. (2021) *El presupuesto de 2021: gastando como si ya no hubiera pandemia.* Mexico City: Mexicanos contra la corrupción y la impunidad.

McKee, M., Gilmore, A.B. and Schwalbe, N. (2005) 'International cooperation and health. Part 1. Issues and concepts', *Journal of Epidemiology and Community Health*, 59, pp. 628–631.

Mercer, T. and Salit, M. (2021) 'Testing at scale during the COVID-19 pandemic', *Nature Reviews Genetics*, 22, pp. 415–426.

Milenio (2020) 'Aplicar más pruebas no garantiza control de COVID-19, afirma López-Gatell', *Milenio*, 10 June. [Online]. Available at: www.milenio.com/videos/politica/aplicar-pruebas-garantiza-control-covid-19-afirma-lopez-gatell (Accessed 15 June 2020).

Morales Fajardo, M.E. and Cadena Inostroza, C. (2020) '(Des)organizando la (des)gobernanza en tiempos de pandemia', *Notas de coyuntura del CRIM (6)*, 5 May, pp. 1–4. Available at: https://ru.crim.unam.mx/handle/123456789/83.

Morawska, L. and Milton, D.K. (2020) 'It is time to address airborne transmission of coronavirus disease 2019 (COVID-19)', *Clinical Infectious Diseases*, 71(9), pp. 2311–2313.

Morin, J.-F. (2014) 'Paradigm shift in the global IP regime: the agency of academics', *Review of International Political Economy*, 21(2), pp. 275–309.

Navarro, M.F. (2020) 'Obligar uso de cubrebocas pone en riesgo derechos humanos: López-Gatell', *Forbes*, 12 August. [Online]. Available at: www.forbes.com.mx/politica-obligar-cubrebocas-riesgo-derechos-humanos-lopez-gatell/ (Accessed 15 August 2020).

Niel, D.M. (2021) 'Fauci on what working for Trump was really like', *New York Times*, 24 January. [Online]. Available at: www.nytimes.com/2021/01/24/health/fauci-trump-covid.html (Accessed 15 June 2021).

Otto, B. *et al.* (2020) *Agua: el aliado clave en la lucha contra el coronavirus.* Mexico: WRI Mexico.

Oxford University (2020) *Our world in data—coronavirus pandemic.* Available at: https://ourworldindata.org/coronavirus (Accessed 25 March 2022).

Pavon, A. (2020) 'No está científicamente demostrado que cubrebocas evite el contagio de COVID-19: AMLO', *SDP noticias*, 24 July. [Online]. Available at: www.sdpnoticias.com/nacional/amlo-no-esta-cientificamente-comprobado-cubrebocas-ayude-contagios-coronavirus-Covid-19.html (Accessed 26 January 2021).

Payne, A. (1953) 'The influenza programme of WHO', *Bulletin World Health Organization*, 8, pp. 755–774.

Perusquia, C. (2020) 'Considera AMLO "autoritario" hacer obligatorio el uso de cubrebocas', *AM Queretaro*, 16 November. [Online]. Available at: https://amque-retaro.com/queretaro/2020/11/16/considera-amlo-autoritario-hacer-obligatorio-el-uso-de-cubrebocas/ (Accessed 15 December 2020).

Petersen, I.H. (2016) 'Facilitators and obstacles to cooperation in international development networks: a network approach', *Development in Practice*, 26(3), pp. 360–374.

Presidencia de la Republica Gobierno de Mexico (2020) *Versión estenográfica de la conferencia de prensa matutina*. Mexico City. [Online]. Available at: www.gob.mx/presidencia (Accessed 5 January 2024).

Public Safety Canada (2012) *North America plan for animal and pandemic influenza (NAPAPI)*. Ottawa: Public Safety Canada. Available at: https://www.publicsafety.gc.ca/cnt/rsrcs/pblctns/nml-pndmc-nflnz/nml-pndmc-nflnz-eng.pdf.

Raustiala, K. (2002) 'The architecture for international cooperation: transgovernmental networks and the future of international law', *Virginia Journal of International Law*, 43(1), p. 1.

Redaccion Animal Político (2020) 'López-Gatell pide a medios difundir uso de cubrebocas, luego de decir que no era eficaz', *Animal Político*, 18 November. [Online]. Available at: www.animalpolitico.com/2020/11/lopez-gatell-medios-difundir-uso-cubrebocas (Accessed 5 September 2020).

Redaccion Aristegui Noticias (2020) 'López-Gatell, nuevo miembro del comité de expertos de la OMS', *Aristegui Noticias*, 12 June. [Online]. Available at: https://aristeguinoticias.com/1206/mexico/lopez-gatell-nuevo-miembro-del-comite-de-expertos-de-la-oms/ (Accessed 5 September 2020).

Ribhi Shawar, Y. (2016) *The impact of internal characteristics on global health epistemic community effectiveness: the cases of global surgery, early childhood development and urban health*. Washington, DC: American University.

Robles de la Rosa, L. (2020) 'No más pruebas, 'es desperdicio de tiempo y recursos': López-Gatell', *Excelsior*, 28 May. [Online]. Available at: No más pruebas, 'es desperdicio de tiempo y recursos': López-Gatell (excelsior.com.mx) (Accessed 15 June 2020).

Rosenthal, P.J. (2020) 'The importance of diagnostic testing during a viral pandemic: early lessons from novel coronavirus disease (COVID-19)', *The American Journal of Tropical Medicine and Hygiene*, 102(5), pp. 915–916.

Ruggie, J. (1998) *Constructing the world polity: essays on international institutionalization*. London: Routledge.

Sebenius, J.K. (1992) 'Challenging conventional explanations of international cooperation: negotiation analysis and the case of epistemic communities', *International Organization*, 46(1), pp. 323–365.

Secretaria de Gobernación México (2020) 'Acuerdo por el que el Consejo de Salubridad General reconoce la epidemia de enfermedad por virus SARS-CoV2 en México, como una enfermedad grave de atención prioritaria, así como se establecen las actividades de preparación y respuesta ante dicha epidemia', *Diario Oficial de la Federación*, 19 marzo.

Secretaria de Salud Mexico (2020) *Se reúne de forma extraordinaria el Comité Nacional para la Seguridad en Salud*. Mexico City: Gobierno de Mexico. [Online]. Available at: www.gob.mx/salud/prensa/se-reune-de-forma-extraordinaria-el-comite-nacional-para-la-seguridad-en-salud?%20idiom=es (Accessed 26 January 2021).

Sending, O.J. (2019) 'Knowledge networks, scientific communities, and evidence-informed policy', in Stone, D. and Maloney, K. (eds.) *The Oxford handbook of global policy and transnational administration*. Oxford: Oxford University Press, pp. 383–400.

Skogstad, G. (2003) 'Legitimacy and policy effectiveness? Network governance and GMO regulation in the European Union', *Journal of European Public Policy*, 10(3), pp. 323–327.

Spath, K. (2005) 'Inside global governance: new borders of a concept', in Lederer, M. and Muller, P. (eds.) *Criticizing global governance*. s.l.: Palgrave Macmillan, pp. 21–44.

Stevens, A. (2007) 'Survival of the ideas that fit: an evolutionary analogy for the use of evidence in policy', *Social Policy and Society*, 6(1), pp. 25–35.

Stone, D. (2008) 'Global public policy, transnational policy communities, and their networks', *The Policy Studies Journal*, 36(1), pp. 19–38.

Stone, D. (2012) 'Transfer and translation of policy', *Policy Studies*, 33(6), pp. 483–499.

Stone, D. and Ladi, S. (2015) 'Global public policy and transnational administration', *Public Administration*, 93(4), pp. 839–855.

Underdal, A. (1998) 'Explaining compliance and defection: three models', *European Journal of International Relations*, 4(1), pp. 5–30.

United Nations Information Centre (2020) 'UNCC Mexico interview with Cristian Morales', 24 March. [Online]. Available at: www.infobioquimica.com/new/2020/03/30/entrevista-a-cristian-morales-representante-de-la-ops-oms-en-mexico/ (Accessed 15 June 2020).

Vargas-Vázquez, A. *et al.* (2021) 'Unequal impact of structural health determinants and comorbidity on COVID-19 severity', *The Journals of Gerontology*, 76(3), pp. e52–e59.

Vergara, R. (2020) 'López-Gatell prevé aumento de casos sospechosos de COVID-19 por presentar un solo síntoma accesorio', *Proceso*, 24 August. [Online]. Available at: www.proceso.com.mx/nacional/2020/8/24/lopez-gatell-preve-aumento-de-casos-sospechosos-de-covid-19-por-presentar-un-solo-sintoma-accesorio-248231.html (Accessed 30 August 2020).

Weiss, S. (2020) 'Mexico is as bad as Brazil in its fight against the pandemic', *Mexico*, 16 August. [Online]. Available at: www.dw.com/es/m%C3%A9xico-est%C3%A1-tan-mal-como-brasil-en-su-lucha-contra-la-pandemia/a-54586633 (Accessed 30 August 2020).

Weiss, T.G., Carayannis, T. and Jolly, R. (2009) 'The third United Nations', *Global Governance*, 15(1), pp. 123–142.

Wendt, A. (1992) 'Anarchy is what states make of it: the social construction of power politics', *International Organization*, 46(2), pp. 391–425.

Weyland, K. (2006) 'The puzzle of policy diffusion', in *Bounded rationality and policy diffusion: social sector reform in Latin America*. Princeton: Princeton University Press, pp. 1–29.

The WHO MERS-CoV Research Group (2013) 'State of knowledge and data gaps of middle east respiratory syndrome coronavirus (MERS-CoV) in humans', *PLoS Currents*, 5. https://doi.org/10.1371/currents.outbreaks.0bf719e352e7478f8ad85fa30127ddb8.

World Health Organization (2000) *A framework for global outbreak alert and response*. Geneva: WHO.

World Health Organization (2008) *International health regulations 2005*. 2nd edn. Geneva: World Health Organization.

World Health Organization (2011a) *A64/10 review committee IHR, report of the review committee on the functioning of the international health regulations (2005) in relation to pandemic (H1N1) 2009*. Geneva: World Health Organization.

World Health Organization (2011b) *Report of the review committee on the functioning of the international health regulations (2005) about pandemic influenza (H1N1) 2009, A64/105*. Geneva: WHO.

World Health Organization (2013) 'Middle east respiratory syndrome coronavirus (MERS-CoV)—update'. Available at: www.who.int/csr/don/2013_06_26/en/ (Accessed 17 April 2018).

World Health Organization (2018) *WHO consultation on MERS CoV clinical trial design*. Geneva: WHO.

World Health Organization (2019, March 28) *WHO collaborative multi-centre research project on severe acute respiratory syndrome (SARS) diagnosis*. [Online]. Available at: https://www.who.int/csr/sars/project/en/ (Accessed 10 September 2020).

World Health Organization (2020a, 5 June) *Advice on the use of masks in the context of COVID-19*. Geneva: WHO.

World Health Organization (2020b, 30 March) *COVID-19—virtual press conference*. WHO. [Online]. Available at: www.who.int/docs/default-source/coronaviruse/ transcripts/who-audio-emergencies-coronavirus-press-conference-full-30mar2020. pdf?sfvrsn=6b68bc4a2 (Accessed 13 January 2024).

World Health Organization (2020c) *Public health criteria to adjust public health measures and social measures in the context of COVID-19*. Geneva: WHO.

World Health Organization (2020d, 30 January) *Statement on the second meeting of the international health regulations (2005) emergency committee regarding the outbreak of novel coronavirus (2019-nCoV)*. WHO. [Online]. Available at: www. who.int/news/item/30-01-2020-statement-on-the-second-meeting-of-the-internati onal-health-regulations-(2005)-emergency-committee-regarding-the-outbreak-of- novel-coronavirus-(2019-ncov) (Accessed 15 December 2021).

World Health Organization (2020e) *WHO coronavirus disease (COVID-19) dashboard with vaccination data*. Geneva: WHO. Available at: https://covid19.who.int/ region/amro/country/mx (Accessed 15 December 2021).

World Health Organization (2020f) *WHO COVID-19 reference laboratory network*. Geneva: WHO. [Online]. Available at: www.who.int/publications/m/item/ who-reference-laboratories-providing-confirmatory-testing-for-covid-19 (Accessed 15 May 2021).

World Health Organization (2020g) *WHO director-general's opening remarks at the media briefing on COVID-19*. WHO. 11 March. [Online]. Available at: www. who.int/director-general/speeches/detail/who-director-general-s-opening-remarks- at-the-media-briefing-on-covid-19-11-march-2020#:~:text=Describing%20 the%20situation%20as%20a,pandemic%20caused%20by%20a%20coronavirus (Accessed 15 December 2020).

World Health Organization (2020h) *Status of collection of assessed contributions, including member states in arrears in the payment of their contributions to an extent that would justify invoking article 7 of the constitution, Res A72/23*. Geneva: WHO, p. 8.

World Health Organization (2021a, June) *WHO recommendations for national SARS-CoV-2 testing strategies and diagnostic capacities, interim guidance*. Geneva: WHO.

World Health Organization (2021b, February) *Contact tracing in the context of COVID-19, interim guidance*. Geneva: WHO.

World Health Organization (2021c) *Global outbreak alert and response network, global meeting*. Geneva: WHO.

World Health Organization (2022) *Networks, committees, advisory groups and task-forces*. Geneva: WHO. [Online]. Available at: www.who.int/groups (Accessed 15 March 2022).

World Health Organization Multicentre Collaborative Network for Severe Acute Respiratory Syndrome (SARS) Diagnosis (2003) 'A multicentre collaboration to investigate the cause of severe acute respiratory syndrome', *The Lancet*, 361(1), pp. 1730–1733.

Worldometers (2022) *Coronavirus*. [Online]. Available at: www.worldometers.info/coronavirus/ (Accessed 22 January 2022).

Youde, J. (2005) 'The development of a counter-epistemic community: AIDS, South Africa, and international regimes', *International Relations*, 19(4), pp. 421–439.

Youde, J. (2011) 'Mediating risk through the international health regulations and bio-political surveillance', *Political Studies*, 59(4), pp. 813–830.

Zacher, M.W. and Keefe, T.J. (2007) *The politics of global health governance. United by contagion*. New York: Palgrave Macmillan.

Zito, A. (2018) 'Instrument constituencies and epistemic community theory', *Policy and Society*, 37(1).

4 The Pernicious Impact of Pandemic Politics

Mexico's Experience With COVID-19 Vaccine Governance

Thomas Legler

Introduction: Explaining the Mexican COVID-19 Vaccination Experience

Four years after the outbreak of the COVID-19 pandemic, it was clear that Mexico's vaccination of its population was problematic. On the positive side, in December 2020, the country held the honour of being the first Latin American country to commence the immunisation of its citizens. On the negative side, especially during the crucial first year of the national vaccination drive in 2021, Mexican authorities were criticised for the slow roll-out of vaccines (Kane Jiménez and Gandy, 2021; Sánchez Talanquer and Sepúlveda, 2024). Critics also highlighted the substantial delay in making shots available for children under 15 years of age (Díaz, 2022; García, 2023; Kane Jiménez and Gandy, 2021; Sánchez Talanquer and Sepúlveda, 2024). It was not until April 2022 that President López Obrador announced that children aged 12 and older would be vaccinated, and until June of that year for those between five and 11. It is also noteworthy that problems with vaccine roll-out have been linked to gross disparities in COVID-19 deaths in states like Chiapas and Puebla, as well as the country's notoriety as the place with the highest number of deaths among health workers in the world: 4,843 (Dávila, 2023; Sánchez Talanquer and Sepúlveda, 2024, p. 278).

Mexico's vaccination statistics are most telling. As Figures 4.1 and 4.2 indicate further ahead in this chapter, in January 2024, Mexico's vaccination rate per 100 population was 175, just above the Latin American average of 160.46 but inferior to 11 other countries in the region. As a share of the population, by March 2023, roughly 76% of Mexicans had received at least one shot, and 64% had acquired all recommended doses. These numbers put Mexico just above the Latin American and world averages, but well below the rates for many other Latin American countries, high-income countries, and upper middle-income countries.[1]

What explains Mexico's suboptimal COVID-19 vaccination performance? After all, objectively speaking, as an upper middle-income country, it arguably possessed the resources and capabilities both to produce its own vaccines and to import an adequate supply. To be fair, it must be mentioned that

DOI: 10.4324/9781003494959-4

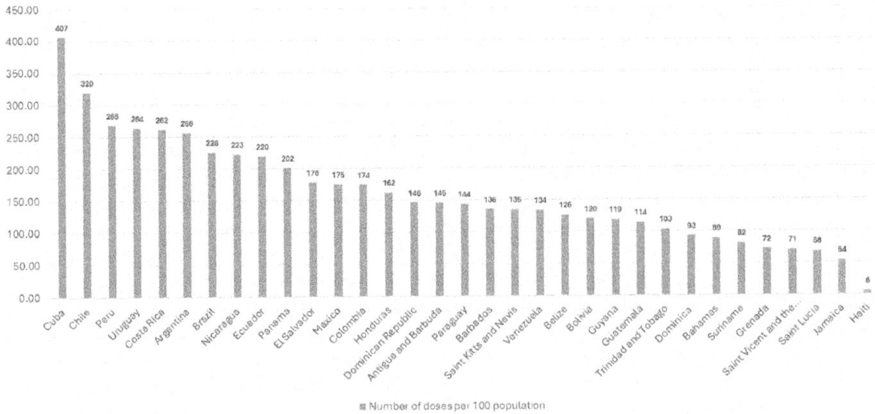

Figure 4.1 Number of COVID-19 vaccination doses per 100 population administered in Latin America and the Caribbean as of January 5, 2024, by country

Source: Statista 2024 COVID-19 vaccination rate by country Latin America 2024 | Statista

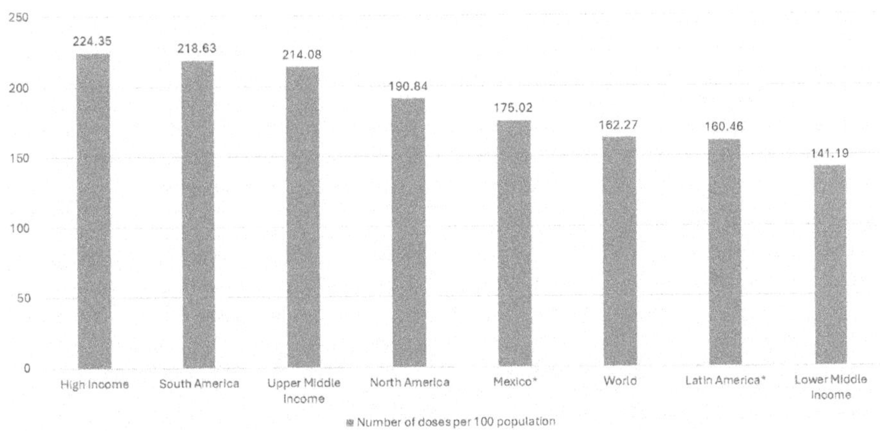

Figure 4.2 Rate of COVID-19 vaccine doses administered worldwide as of March 20, 2023, by select country, territory, or region

Source: Statista 2024 COVID-19 vaccination rate by country Latin America 2024 | Statista Countries with highest COVID vaccination dose rates 2023 | Statista

Mexico and the rest of the planet were confronted with the unprecedented, urgent, and enormous challenges entailed in filling in the governance gaps required in order to produce, distribute, and apply vast quantities of vaccines in record time. As I shall discuss in the following pages, global vaccine governance and the Mexican government response had to be constructed at a frantic pace and largely from scratch. In keeping with the central theme of this volume, I argue that Mexico's problematic experience with COVID-19 vaccines has to do with two particular deleterious types of pandemic politics that came together in the meeting of governance and government: an adverse global political economy and a harmful Mexican vaccine populism.

The following analysis is divided broadly into two parts. The first half of the chapter examines the global governance side of Mexico's experience with COVID-19 vaccines. It sketches the evolution of the global vaccine governance complex prior to and during the pandemic and links it to a detrimental global political economy for pandemic vaccines. The inadequacy of the newly created COVAX vaccine mechanism created an urgent imperative for Mexican authorities to source the country's vaccine requirements through a pragmatic combination of bilateral contracts with multinational pharmaceutical companies and donations from governments of the Global North caught up in a geopolitical rivalry. In the second half, I evaluate how the populist political tendencies of the Mexican government hurt the country's vaccination effort. The country's centralised and politicised vaccination drive caused unnecessary delays in the crucial first year of the roll-out and made certain segments of the population vulnerable to infection.

The Rise of the Global Pandemic Vaccine Governance Complex

In order to understand fully the Mexican experience, it is important first to appreciate what transpired with global pandemic vaccine governance, both before and during the COVID-19 pandemic. This section sketches the evolution of a global pandemic vaccine governance complex against the backdrop of a series of outbreaks that occurred during the first two decades of the 21st century and prior to the COVID-19 crisis. It starts by presenting a brief overview of the relevant literature and defining the key concept of global governance complex (GGC). It then identifies the core institutions that would come to comprise the GGC for pandemic vaccines. Importantly, with the benefit of hindsight, it is possible to see that there were already worrisome signs of things to come in terms of the global political economy of vaccine governance and its potential effects on the access of countries like Mexico to vaccines in the event of a pandemic.

The study of global governance processes has undergone a metamorphosis since the concept was first invented and popularised by the Commission on Global Governance (1995) during the 1990s. From an initial focus on the role of individual actors, institutions, organisations, and regimes, scholars have increasingly recognised the growing proliferation, interconnection, overlap, and hierarchical relations among these elements in the governance of specific global or regional issue-areas or problems. Accordingly, governance thinkers have been prompted to capture this increasing complexity in new conceptual development. In this regard, various authors began to refer to governance architectures as "the overarching system of public and private institutions that are valid or active in a given issue area of world politics. These architectures comprise organizations, regimes, and other forms of principles, norms, regulations, and decision-making procedures" (Biermann *et al.*, 2009, p. 15). Concurrently, others developed the notion of regime complex, defined as "a set of overlapping and perhaps even contradictory regimes that share a common focus" (Alter and Raustiala, 2018. p. 330; see also Alter and Meunier, 2009; Orsini, Morin and Young, 2013; Raustiala, 2004).

The most recent addition to the conceptual toolkit for studying governance complexity is the concept of GGC. GGCs are "clusters of overlapping institutions and actors that govern specific policy issues" (Eilstrup-Sangiovanni and Westerwinter (2022, p. 233). Eilstrup-Sangiovanni and Westerwinter also note that a GGC is "a system of formally separate institutions whose memberships, mandates or functions overlap, but that operate in the absence of a formal authority empowered to resolve rule conflicts (2022, p. 236). Moreover, a GGC comprises "a system of governance composed of at least three international or transnational institutions or actors whose mandates, functions and memberships overlap, and that jointly address a specific policy problem" (Eilstrup-Sangiovanni and Westerwinter, 2022, p. 238). Building on the emphasis of international institutional proliferation, overlap, and complexity found in the concepts of governance architecture and regime complexes, the advantage of the new term is that it adds networks of actors to the equation, as well as their diversity and hierarchical interactions.

During the first decades of this century, a GGC in the area of pandemic vaccines began to take shape following a series of pandemics that had occurred, including the 2003 SARS virus, the 2006 H5N1 or bird flu virus, the 2009 H1N1 virus, and the 2014–2015 Ebola virus. As I sketch in the following pages, over time, this complex would grow to encompass extensive global networks of state, intergovernmental, private, and transnational actors; a vaccine research, development, financing, procurement, and distribution ecosystem; and a corresponding normative structure. Anchored in a set of public-private partnerships (PPPs), this architecture comprised four institutional pillars: a growing role for the World Health Organization (WHO) in terms of norm promotion and governance orchestration; vaccine procurement; pandemic virus data sharing; and a mechanism for funding vaccine research and development.

First, the WHO assumed a growing coordination and orchestration role for global vaccine governance during the new millennium.[2] In 1999, the WHO established the Strategic Advisory Group of Experts on Immunisation to guide its involvement in vaccine-related activities. Although the 2005 International Health Regulations (IHR) (World Health Organization, 2005) did not define clear prerogatives for the WHO with respect to pandemic vaccine development, production, and distribution, it did empower the organisation in a broader sense to assume a crucial coordinating and normative function in terms of pandemic preparedness and response against PHEIC. This would serve as the basis for the organisation to expand its pandemic vaccine governance mandates over the coming years. The IHR did reinforce the WHO's responsibility for the approval of new vaccines.

Through a series of instruments, the WHO gradually expanded its orchestration role *vis-à-vis* the extensive universe of governmental, non-governmental, private, and academic actors involved as stakeholders in the promotion of vaccines as a crucial strategy against epidemics and pandemics. In 2006, it launched a ten-year plan called the Global Action Plan for Influenza Vaccines, or GAP (World Health Organization, 2006). Importantly, GAP recognised the need to overcome inequitable access to pandemic influenza vaccines, to create and store adequate global supplies of vaccines against pandemics, and to strengthen technology transfer and production capacity among low- and middle-income countries.

The 2009 H1N1 pandemic catalysed the expansion of the WHO's role in the influenza vaccine field. The WHO led the first ever coordinated global vaccine response to a pandemic virus through the creation of the temporary Pandemic Influenza A (H1N1) Vaccine Deployment Initiative. Under the coordination of the WHO, this PPP managed to mobilise extensive resources among its state, intergovernmental, non-governmental, philanthropic, and corporate partners in order to donate and deliver approximately 78 million doses of pandemic H1N1 vaccines to vulnerable populations around the globe (World Health Organization, 2012). The WHO also fulfilled an important role in vaccine pre-qualification and approval, especially for poorer countries with limited domestic capacity for these activities.

Drawing on the lessons learnt from the 2006 H5N1 bird flu outbreak and the 2009 H1N1 pandemic, in 2011, the WHO (World Health Organization, 2011) launched the Pandemic Influenza Preparedness Framework (PIP Framework). The PIP Framework was a dual-purpose instrument: to facilitate the rapid and timely sharing of influenza virus data between their countries of origin, often from the Global South, and vaccine developers concentrated in the Global North; and to strengthen global access to influenza vaccines. It sought to overcome the recent controversy surrounding the government of Indonesia's refusal to share samples of the bird flu H5N1 virus from the 2006 outbreak. That is, the latter's resistance was on the grounds that developing countries received little or no benefit when pharmaceutical companies used them for vaccine or medicine patent development and commercial gain.

Importantly, the PIP Framework committed pharmaceutical countries to cover half the annual costs of the WHO's Global Influenza Surveillance and Response System in exchange for access to genetic sequence data for pandemic influenza viruses from developing countries. The Framework also extended the WHO's pandemic preparedness and response authority to include a growing coordinating role in areas such as vaccine development, production, and stockpiling. The PIP Framework also highlighted the WHO's expanding normative function in areas such as the promotion of virus sharing, tiered pricing, and technology transfer in the interest of enhancing the access of developing countries to pandemic vaccines.

In 2016, the WHO created the R&D Blueprint on the basis of what it had learnt facilitating the development of medical products in the context of the

Ebola outbreak. This was a global strategy and preparedness plan whose purpose was to offer detailed roadmaps for specific infectious diseases in order to foster the rapid activation of research and development activities for diagnostics, treatments, and vaccines in the event of an epidemic. The R&D Blueprint resulted in the rapid development of the first ever effective vaccine against Ebola (Kieny and Salama, 2017).

Finally, shortly before the onset of the COVID-19 pandemic, the WHO unveiled its 2019–2030 Global Influenza Strategy (see World Health Organization, 2019). The Strategy recognised the need to prioritise and strengthen pandemic vaccine response capacity in light of the recent experience with serious outbreaks such as the 2009 H1N1 virus and the 2014–2015 West African Ebola epidemic and out of a growing concern for potential future global pandemics. It prioritised vaccine research and development, recognising vaccination as the best tool in the fight against influenza. It advocated global vaccine preparedness plans for switching rapidly from seasonal to pandemic vaccine manufacturing in the event of an influenza health emergency. Finally, it called for the continuation of industry and civil society support for the aforementioned PIP Framework as the means to promote more equitable access to vaccines and antiviral drugs.

The development of an institutional mechanism for vaccine procurement and delivery at accessible prices was a second crucial pillar in the emerging vaccine governance complex. In 1999, a coalition of public and private partners established the Global Alliance for Vaccines and Immunization (GAVI), the Vaccine Alliance (see McNeill and Sandberg, 2014; Sandberg, Andresen and Bjune, 2010). With substantial start-up funding from the Gates Foundation, GAVI is a PPP whose partners include the WHO, UNICEF, the World Bank, as well as governments, industry, academics, and others. Through its Advanced Market Mechanism and partners, it has sought to reduce prices for the procurement of routine vaccines. Although its original mandate was to increase low-income countries' access to children's vaccines, this was expanded to include pandemic vaccines in the context of the Ebola crisis. It would subsequently become a key player in the COVAX mechanism that arose during the COVID-19 pandemic (de Bengy Puyvallée, 2024).

The third pillar was an open access platform for the sharing of infectious disease data to foster vaccine development. Motivated by the obstacles for data sharing that were present during the 2006 avian influenza outbreak mentioned earlier, in 2008, GISAID, the Global Initiative on Sharing All Influenza Data, was established for this purpose. This PPP and the EpiFlu database that it had developed with the financial support of the German government and private donors were soon called into action during the 2009 A(H1N1) pandemic. The GISAID's data sharing model had the potential to expand its applicability over time beyond influenza viruses to include other pathogens with pandemic potential (Shu and McCauley, 2017).

The fourth pillar to arise was a global architecture for funding vaccine-related research. One such financing mechanism for timely vaccine development against emerging infectious diseases was the Global Research Collaboration for Infectious Disease Preparedness (GloPID-R). Glopid-R was established in 2013 as a global network and coalition of 32-member research funding organisations and ten observers that set themselves the goals of promoting rapid research responses to and data sharing during public health emergencies with pandemic potential. This entity cut its teeth on the 2015 Zika outbreak, which it used as the basis for developing readiness plans for future contagious disease incidents (Matthiessen *et al.*, 2016).

Another financing mechanism, the Coalition for Epidemic Preparedness Innovations, or CEPI, was created in 2017 in response to the Ebola epidemic in 2014–2015. CEPI is a PPP that pools the resources of public, private, non-governmental, and academic stakeholders (Brende *et al.*, 2017) and whose mission is to foster rapid vaccine development and equitable access to vaccines against diseases with epidemic potential, especially in poorer countries of the Global South where market incentives are weak (Brende *et al.*, 2017; Gouglas *et al.*, 2019; Huneycutt *et al.*, 2020). Prior to the COVID-19 pandemic, CEPI funded vaccine research against pathogens such as Lassa, Nipah, MERS, and Chikungunya.

In sum, on the eve of the COVID-19 pandemic, the rudimentary elements of a global pandemic vaccine governance complex existed: the WHO as a central coordinating and orchestration agent as well as institutional mechanisms for vaccine procurement, data sharing, research and development, and financing. Overall, the main institutional scaffolding for the complex was provided by the creation of a series of interlocking PPPs (de Bengy Puyvallée, 2024). The WHO, GAVI, GISAID, GLOPID-R, and CEPI were also in the vanguard of efforts to promote a set of norms concerning vaccine governance, among others: the promotion of vaccines as the best antidote against pandemics; affordable access for poorer countries to vaccines; virus data sharing; vaccine stockpiling; vaccine technology transfer; and the enhancement of production capacity in the Global South.

This governance complex already displayed tensions and contradictions before the COVID-19 outbreak. Importantly, despite the rhetorical claims of the WHO and other actors that comprised the growing number of PPPs to promote vaccine equity, the aforementioned architecture was a reflection of international market-driven vaccine development, production, and distribution that relied on private pharmaceutical suppliers. It was also rife with potential North-South disparities and tensions. Profitability considerations meant that multinational pharmaceutical companies that were largely concentrated in northern countries often had little interest or incentive in developing or distributing vaccines against infectious diseases for poor countries in the Global South. The emerging pandemic vaccine governance complex also overlapped with the global intellectual property regime, such that any efforts to promote global vaccine equity would have to contend with the jealous protection of intellectual secrets by these companies. Despite the widespread rhetoric of the need to promote global access to vaccines, there already was evidence from the 2009 H1N1 pandemic that wealthier countries with superior manufacturing capacity and purchasing power were prepared to engage in the practice of stockpiling copious supplies of vaccines at the expense of the access of poorer countries (Bollyky and Bown, 2020a, pp. 100–101). These problems would prove to have serious consequences for countries like Mexico during the COVID-19 crisis.

The Global Political Economy of COVID-19 Governance: Against Vaccine Equity

The limited global vaccine architecture that existed at the outset of the outbreak left governance actors scrambling to fill in the governance gaps[3] that impeded the rapid development, production, distribution, and delivery of effective and affordable vaccines against the virus. It is a credit to the efforts of these stakeholders that the first vaccines were developed, approved, distributed, and applied within less than a year of the initial declaration by the WHO of the outbreak as a PHEIC on January 20, 2020. During 2021, some 8.7 billion vaccine doses were administered around the world as part of the largest and fastest vaccination drive in history (Theil, 2021).

However, this section underlines that the particular pandemic politics that unfolded were not conducive to offering many middle- and low-income countries like Mexico ready and equitable access to the precious new vaccines. The prevalent global political economy of pandemic vaccine governance favoured the control of vaccine development, stock, and distribution by the governments and pharmaceutical companies of the Global North and prevented COVID-19 vaccinations from becoming a truly global public good. Instead, the mix of the global governance and political economy of vaccines produced winners and losers along North-South lines. Countries like Mexico were left facing an urgent imperative for pragmatism: to adopt the measures necessary in order to obtain an adequate supply of vaccines for their populations.

During the first six months of the COVID-19 pandemic, there were promising signs that global health cooperation and solidarity could attain unprecedented heights. In April 2020, in a pair of historic resolutions, members of the United Nations General Assembly (2020a, 2020b) recognised the urgency for and essentiality of global solidarity, unity, and reinvigorated multilateral cooperation, as well as fair and equitable global access to medicines, vaccines, and medical equipment. These calls were echoed during the World Health Assembly (WHA) that was held in May 2020. However, the WHA went even farther in its resolution WHA73.1 in recognising extensive immunisation against COVID-19 as a *global public good* (World Health Assembly, 2020).

With respect to vaccine governance, the response to COVID-19 entailed both the recourse to and retooling of existing institutional mechanisms as well as the creation of new architecture. For example, the WHO activated its pre-existing R&D Blueprint in an attempt to kickstart the rapid development of tests, treatments, and vaccines. From its earlier focus on influenza strains, GISAID expanded its mandate to become the global repository for genetic sequence data for this coronavirus (Lurie, Keusch and Dzau, 2021).

In April 2020, the WHO and its partners GAVI and CEPI established the ambitious Access to COVID-19 Tools Accelerator (ACT-A), a PPP whose purpose was to speed up the development and promote the equitable distribution of three crucial aids to combat the pandemic: diagnostics, treatments, and vaccines. In June 2020, the vaccine arm of ACT-A was formally launched: COVAX. With a specific focus on the rapid development, production, procurement, and equitable access to COVID-19 vaccines, COVAX was the brainchild of GAVI and CEPI, with support from the WHO and UNICEF. As a "super public-private partnership" (Storeng, de Bengy Puyvallée and Stein, 2023), COVAX was intended to be a powerful buyers' pool (Yamey *et al.*, 2022). According to this pooling logic, participating governments would collectively channel their financial resources through COVAX, which would enable this mechanism to fund vaccine research, development, and manufacturing, as well as reduce the cost of vaccines through large collective purchases from pharmaceutical suppliers.

In May 2020, the WHO and the government of Costa Rica, in partnership with the UNDP, the Medicines Patent Pool, the UN Technology Bank, and Unitaid, created the COVID-19 Technology Access Pool (C-TAP). C-TAP was a multilateral global pooling mechanism to facilitate the sharing of intellectual property, knowledge, and data on a voluntary basis in order to propel the development of COVID-19-related health products, including vaccines (Geiger and McMahon, 2021).

This global pandemic vaccine governance complex could boast some impressive achievements. Never before had there been such a dramatic and rapid development, production, and administering of vaccines: ten billion doses in less than one and a half years (Yadav, 2021). By December 2023, more than 13 billion doses of the COVID-19 vaccine had been administered globally (WHO, 2023). The COVAX facility became the largest vaccine procurement and supply operation in history, with approximately two billion vaccines and safe injection devices shipped to 146 economies before its closure in December 2023 (www.gavi.org/covax/).

Nonetheless, the disparities in access to COVID-19 vaccines and vaccination were appalling, especially in the crucial first year and a half of roll-out. Whereas 76%–78% of people in upper-middle- and high-income countries had enjoyed at least one dose by the end of 2021, this figure was only 8.5% of people in low-income countries (de Bengy Puyvallée and Storeng, 2022, p. 2). COVAX, on which the majority of poor countries originally relied for their vaccine supply, failed to deliver even half of its targeted two billion doses for 2021, the crucial initial year of vaccination. Instead of establishing itself as the anchor for global COVID-19 vaccination, COVAX supplied only a fraction of the 9.25 billion doses that were administered globally in 2021 (de Bengy Puyvallée and Storeng, 2022). The WHO failed to reach its target of inoculating 70% of people in all countries by mid-2022 (WHO, 2021).

The gross vaccine inequity that prevailed in 2021 led the heads of the International Monetary Fund, WHO, World Bank Group, and the World Trade Organization to label the situation as a "two-track pandemic": one in which wealthy countries enjoyed access and poorer ones were left behind (Georgieva *et al.*, 2021). The WHO's Director-General, Tedros Adhanom Ghebreyesus, described the situation as "vaccine apartheid" (Reuters, 2021).

The rhetorical recognition and aspiration in the World Health Assembly's historic resolution WHA73.1 of the need to promote vaccination against COVID-19 as a global public good was not achieved in reality. Global vaccine governance failed to satisfy the two defining characteristics of any public good: non-rivalry—each individual's consumption of a good does not subtract from that of another individual (and vice versa); and non-excludability—the impossibility of excluding any individual from consuming the good. Instead, as King Mantilla and Carranza Barona (2022) observed, COVID-19 vaccines became a prime example of the commodification of health.

Powerful global political economy tendencies distorted vaccine governance in at least four important and interconnected ways: the design of governance institutions; the defence of intellectual property; vaccine nationalism and regionalism; and vaccine diplomacy. First, the institutional preference for PPPs to anchor vaccine governance would prove to be an important source of mal governance. Countries and pharmaceutical companies of the Global North that already enjoyed virtual monopoly control over the research, development, and production of vaccines saw their influence enhanced via PPPs. Despite ample rhetoric across PPPs such as Gavi, CEPI, and COVAX about the need for vaccine equity, these informal organisations reinforced asymmetries between the Global North and South.

Rather than becoming the exclusive global mechanism for the acquisition and distribution of vaccines on the basis of mandatory participation for all states, COVAX relied on the voluntary commitment of governments. Accordingly, COVAX and other PPPs became governance mechanisms for partially addressing the pandemic challenges of *other people* from the Global South, rather than vaccine globalism (Bollyky and Bown, 2020b). Whereas many resource- and vaccine-poor middle- and low-income countries became reliant on these PPPs for much of their vaccine financing and supply, richer countries on the whole preferred to obtain their supply through direct transactions with pharmaceutical companies. Accordingly, COVAX never achieved its potential as a powerful buyer's pool. Instead, it became an inadvertent defender of the status quo and a vehicle for charity in which a select group of wealthier countries made limited and insufficient donations of vaccines to poorer countries (de Bengy Puyvallée and Storeng, 2022; Krishnan, 2021; Yamey *et al.*, 2022).

The voluntary aspect was also present in the creation of C-TAP. Sadly, this mechanism for pooling patents, knowledge, and data went largely unused. To date, only a handful of research and academic institutions have shared their technologies, and it took until 2023 for the first private pharmaceutical company, Medigen Vaccine Biologics, to make a vaccine available through the platform (Guilbaud, 2023; Venkatesan, 2023).

Second, despite the obvious advantages of the sharing of vaccine data and know-how for combatting the COVID-19 pandemic, as well as massive public investment in vaccine research, COVID-19 vaccines were developed and produced under the existing profit-oriented intellectual property regime connected to the Trade-Related Aspects of Intellectual Property Rights (TRIPS). In May 2021, in an effort to boost global production of and more equitable access to COVID-19 vaccines, President Joe Biden advocated a temporary waiver of the intellectual property protection that companies received under TRIPS. Nevertheless, a powerful set of actors that included pharmaceutical companies, the European Union (EU), and even Bill Gates put up a spirited and successful defence of the intellectual property rights of the companies that had recently developed new vaccines against the coronavirus (Krishnan, 2021).

Although, on the whole, vaccine developers did not share their intellectual property, they benefitted from the free exchange of genome sequences from across the planet. They upheld select crucial knowledge as a private good (patents and intellectual property) rather than a public good (free access to knowledge) (King Mantilla and Carranza Barona, 2022).

Third, COVAX and the promise that it entailed in terms of more equitable vaccine globalism were thwarted by the rise of vaccine nationalism and regionalism. Vaccine nationalism can be defined as a "my country first approach" (Bollyky and Bown, 2020a, pp. 96–97) in which governments prioritise unilaterally the vaccine needs of their own populations over collective efforts to promote international vaccine cooperation, coordination, sharing equity, and vaccines as a global public good.

Vaccine nationalism consisted of various nationalistic measures. The development of vaccines was supported by substantial public funding from countries that later received preferential access to those vaccines through advance purchases (King Mantilla and Carranza Barona, 2022; Yamey *et al.*, 2022), to the detriment of the COVAX mechanism and the access of poorer countries. The bilateral transactions of these governments with pharmaceutical companies were often completed with little transparency, affecting the prices that other countries were able to negotiate. Their hoarding of vaccines and related supplies disrupted crucial global supply chains. In an effort to ensure domestic supply, nationalistic authorities also imposed export controls on their countries' vaccine-related manufactures. The ensuing competitive dynamic drove up prices and impeded the efforts by poorer countries, with limited market power, to access vaccines and associated vaccination materials in a timely manner (Lurie, Keusch and

Dzau, 2021, p. 1233), with adverse consequences for the health of their populations.

Global vaccine governance was also affected by *vaccine regionalism*. In addition to the rampant vaccine nationalism among its individual member states, the EU also hurt vaccine globalism by strengthening its own regional vaccine governance. Instead of prioritising the consolidation of COVAX, EU authorities adopted a series of measures that favoured vaccine development, approval, production, and distribution within the European space at the expense of vaccine globalism (Gratius, Legler and Quezada, 2021). Ironically, the very same EU had been a principal sponsor of the historic World Health Assembly resolution A73 in May 2020 that had advocated for vaccines as a global public good. The EU had also supposedly defended global health multilateralism when President Trump withdrew the US' membership from the WHO, hosting a Global Pledging Summit in June 2020 to raise funds for the new COVAX facility (Guilbaud, 2023, p. 62).

Finally, the pattern of vaccine diplomacy that emerged during the pandemic also hurt global vaccine governance. In the process of developing COVID-19 vaccines, a handful of countries with concentrated economic, industrial, scientific, and pharmaceutical capacities became *vaccine powers*: China, the EU, India, the United Kingdom, and the United States (Yadav, 2021). In their hands, vaccines became a powerful tool not only of commerce but also of diplomacy. In their decisions concerning how and where to donate vaccines, these powers confronted a tension between advancing their own foreign policy goals and strengthening global public health. Sadly, the latter lost out; in its ambition to become the principal global mechanism for vaccine acquisition and distribution, COVAX had to contend with targeted bilateral donations between vaccine-producing countries and recipient countries that were politically more visible and thus more advantageous for foreign policy ends than those that it received (de Bengy Puyvallée and Storeng, 2022). In a context of growing geopolitical rivalry among the United States, the EU, China, and Russia, vaccine donations (along with masks and other medical supplies) became a valuable diplomatic tool with considerable soft power potential. Vaccine diplomacy became part of what has been called the "geopolitics of vaccination" (Malacalza and Fagaburu, 2022). This is the context in which Mexican authorities had to procure an adequate supply of vaccines in record time.

Vaccine Populism in the Mexican Government Response to COVID-19

When it came to the task of organising the mass vaccination of the Mexican population beginning in 2021, the López Obrador government confronted a challenging situation that was not entirely of its own making. The previous section underscored that the adverse global political economy of vaccine governance left countries like Mexico facing a serious vaccine supply bottleneck that impeded ready access to vaccines in the crucial early months of vaccination. By March 2022, COVAX had only managed to supply roughly one-fifth of Mexico's vaccine needs, obliging the government to source the remaining four fifths of its requirements via private contracts or donations in a seller's market (Sánchez Talanquer and Sepúlveda, 2024, p. 248). Moreover, the policies of previous governments had contributed to an historic erosion of domestic vaccine capacity in the country (Valderrama *et al.*, 2021). Finally, an infrastructure for the immunisation of adults did not exist prior to the pandemic and had to be constructed from scratch (Sánchez Talanquer and Sepúlveda, 2024, p. 277).

Notwithstanding these structural impediments, like elsewhere around the planet, Mexican authorities did have decisive agency in terms of determining the course of and outcome of vaccination in the country. As Figure 4.1 illustrates, it is instructive that three years after the commencement of the pandemic, Cuba, Peru, Chile, Uruguay, Costa Rica, Argentina, Brazil, Nicaragua, Ecuador, Panama, and El Salvador (in that order) all had vaccination rates per 100 inhabitants that were superior to Mexico.[4] As Figure 4.2 reveals, Mexico's immunisation statistics were also inferior to the averages for high-income, upper-middle income, North American, and South American countries and only slightly superior to those for the world and Latin America.

Why the difference? Various studies have drawn attention to a global divide in national responses to the COVID-19 pandemic regarding their positive or negative impact on health security and the economy. On one side of the divide, more successful responses were linked to competent public administration, policy informed by scientific evidence, public trust in bureaucracies, and the deference of political leaders to public health professionals and experts. On the other side, populist strongmen personally orchestrated politicised responses that often ran counter to scientific evidence and weakened public health apparatuses rather than strengthen them (see Bayerlein *et al.*, 2021; Hanson and Kopstein, 2021; Lasco, 2020; Sánchez Talanquer and Sepúlveda, 2024, p. 29; Touchton *et al.*, 2023).

As I elaborate later, the Mexican experience with vaccines fits into the latter group. The particular brand of populist vaccine politics goes a long way in explaining the dismal vaccination performance outlined at the beginning of this chapter. In this section, I blame vaccine-related populism for contributing to a vaccination strategy that subscribed more to political than technical and scientific criteria (see also Sánchez Talanquer and Sepúlveda, 2024). This resulted in a relatively slow process of vaccination that left millions of Mexicans unnecessarily unprotected against the virus. It also led to the selective exclusion of and delay in vaccinating certain segments of the population, such as doctors and health workers from private health institutions, children, and people with comorbidities, in spite of the recommendations of international experts. Finally, this harmful type of pandemic politics weakened the public sector at precisely the moment when it needed to be bolstered.

The populist moment (Brubaker, 2017) in Mexico did not arise with the onset of the COVID-19 pandemic. It began in earnest during the 2018 election process that resulted in the victory of presidential candidate Andrés Manuel López Obrador. López Obrador adopted a populist political style and discourse in which he fomented social and political polarisation in the form of a growing antagonistic divide between the people and the corrupt Mexican establishment, which he called alternately *"fifís,"* neoliberals, conservatives, and the *mafia in power.* Thanks to a landslide victory, he positioned himself as the champion and legitimate president of the people, launching a sustained rhetorical attack against the alleged corruption of Mexico's existing political elites and under the rubric of what he labelled the Fourth Transformation, a series of social reforms in favour of the country's poor.

Prior to the pandemic, he did extend his populist-inspired government agenda to the public health sector, dismantling the existing Seguro Popular (Popular Insurance), which he attacked as a neoliberal initiative allegedly rife with corruption and for its exclusion of millions of poor people. With the launch of the successor programme, the Instituto de Salud para el Bienestar (Health Institute for Wellbeing, or INSABI), he committed health authorities to provide free universal health coverage for all Mexicans who lacked social security. As a harbinger of things to come for the country's COVID-19 vaccination, López Obrador dramatically extended health coverage to millions of additional citizens without a corresponding increase in the national public health budget. On the contrary, INSABI was launched in 2019 in the context of the president's commitment to fiscal austerity, or what he preferred calling *republican austerity* (see the chapter by Palacio Ludeña and Velázquez Leyer in this volume).

It is important to acknowledge the idiosyncratic elements of Mexican pre-pandemic populism that carried over to the government's response to COVID-19. President López Obrador combined eclectic and often contradictory elements in his political style, discourse, and agenda: a permanent rhetorical and adversarial campaign against the allegedly corrupt elite establishment of former governments and their allies; the discursive construction of the prior corrupt neoliberal order as the chief culprit for the problems suffered by the country's poor; dramatic increased public spending for select social programmes, such as pensions and scholarships, while promoting republican austerity across the public sector; and nationalism (see Dresser, 2022, 2024; Dussauge-Laguna, 2022).

Just like the overall official response to the pandemic, the López Obrador government's approach to COVID-19 vaccines and vaccination was characterised by strong populist impulses that were consistent with what has been called medical populism. This phenomenon can be defined as a political style based on performances of public health crises that constructs antagonistic relations between "the people" whose lives have been jeopardised by "the (medical) establishment" (Lasco and Curato, 2019, pp. 1–2). According to Lasco and Curato (2019; Lasco, 2020), medical populism rests on three legs:

the application in a health crisis of the populist discursive appeal to the people in opposition to the establishment; the dramatisation and performance of crisis; and discursive simplification.

With respect to the latter, leaders invoke what has been called *epistemological populism*: the recourse to rhetoric that is often anti-intellectual or anti-expert and values the everyday knowledge, life experience, and common sense of "common people" (Brubaker, 2017; Saurette and Gunster, 2011). This discursive trait was captured in a distinct presidential policy narrative that underpinned the government's vaccine initiative (Peci, González and Dussauge-Laguna, 2022). The narrative was marked by the limited, selective, and ambiguous use of scientific evidence, its emphasis on plain talk and that the president and his government had the situation under control, the stoic outlook that risks and threats are a part of life, as well as the need to return to normal life as soon as possible (Peci, González, and Dussauge-Laguna, 2022). Crucially, through his narrative, the president was the chief interpreter, spokesperson, and communicator concerning the pandemic.

Various authors have signalled the deleterious effect that López Obrador's populism has had on the country's policymaking (Dussauge-Laguna, 2022; Renteria and Arellano-Gault, 2021). In line with the analysis of Hanson and Kopstein (2021), President López Obrador embodied the return of patrimonial rule, in which leaders with contempt for public health professionals and experts assumed personal control over health crisis management with the assistance of politically loyal appointees rather than deference to existing competent public health authorities and impersonal rules. Interestingly, these authors offer an important gender observation concerning this patrimonial form of crisis management: López Obrador was part of a pathological global trend of narcissistic, self-serving *male* leaders.

Renteria and Arellano-Gault (2021) refer to *downsizing populism* for the harmful effect of this patrimonial rule on Mexican public administration. That is, in tune with his negative portrayal of the existing state bureaucracy as neoliberal, corrupt, and untrustworthy, López Obrador oversaw tendencies to downsize and weaken the workforce, infrastructure, and institutional capacities of Mexico's public sector, precisely at a moment when the country urgently required strengthened public administration.

Populist influences were felt in Mexico's COVID-19 vaccination strategy in two important, intertwined ways: the centralisation and politicisation of public health authority and processes. First, the centralisation of vaccine-related activity subscribed to the populist logic of establishing unmitigated and direct relations between López Obrador and the people, as manifested in both government institutions and communications.

Institutionally, in the months prior to the beginning of Mexico's vaccination drive, López Obrador neutralised the existing government architecture for the management of public health emergencies that had been codified in Mexican law, the General Health Council (CSG) and the National Health

Council (CNS). In their place, the president imposed a vertical decision-making structure centred on the presidency and the Undersecretariat for Prevention and Health Promotion at the Ministry of Health (Sánchez Talanquer and Sepúlveda, 2024).

Accordingly, government communications with the public were concentrated and personified in two people: President López Obrador and the Undersecretary of Health, Hugo López-Gatell Ramírez. Daily press conferences delivered by these two through the president's morning programme called the *Mañanera* became the mainstay of information for the Mexican population during the pandemic (see Natal, 2021). This structure enabled López Obrador and López-Gatell, "the scientist," to serve as the main interpreters of and government spokespeople for the health crisis, to monopolise the supposed truth, and to control information about the pandemic and the public's access to it.

Centralisation was directly manifested in the government's vaccination programme launched in 2021, Operation Roadrunner. Rather than a joint federal-state undertaking, this initiative would be under the operational command of the Presidency of the Republic with logistical and technical support from the National System of Integral Development for the Family and the Undersecretariat for Prevention and Health Promotion at the Ministry of Health. Instead of building on the existing vaccination architecture that existed through the Universal Vaccination Program or across state and local governments, the López Obrador administration opted to roll out vaccines through the creation and operationalisation of 10,000 brigades that would mount itinerant vaccination centres on the go (Sánchez Talanquer and Sepúlveda, 2024).

This centralisation had important consequences for vaccination performance. The elimination of the responsibility of the CSN and the CNS for crisis management translated into the closure of institutionalised spaces for dialogue with and participation of medical doctors and scientists in decision-making, thereby sacrificing the harnessing of a whole-of-government and whole-of-society approach to crisis management and vaccination. State and local governments were bypassed or underutilised.

On the communication side, centralisation lent itself to the polarisation and antagonisation of public opinion instead of the promotion of dialogue, consensus-building, unity, and coordination. It also led to the silencing or curbing of alternative voices, as well as the control and lack of transparency in information and statistics (Sánchez Talanquer and Sepúlveda, 2024, p. 275).

The marginalisation of scientific and medical experts obliged them to use the media in order to share their health recommendations with the general public and voice their opinions and critiques of government policy. This resulted in the publication or transmission of a flurry of letters, opinion pieces, books, and reports (see, e.g. Frenk and Gómez Dantés, 2021; Infobae,

2021; Moreno, 2022; Sánchez Talanquer *et al.*, 2021; Ximénez Fyvie, 2021, 2022). Accordingly, the government's centralisation drive fuelled a mutually reinforcing and completely unnecessary polarisation between health authorities and experts.

Second, the flipside of centralisation was the politicisation of the vaccination process. From the moment in which the vaccine roll-out process overlapped with the 2021 midterm elections, the government's critics in the scientific and medical community accused it of favouring political over scientific criteria in its vaccine strategy (Díaz, 2022; Redacción, 2023; Moreno, 2022). Mexico's pandemic tsar, Hugo López-Gatell, was attacked for his "pseudo-scientific explanations" and "health dictatorship" (García, 2023).

The epitome of the politicisation of the vaccination process was Operation Roadrunner. Instead of the exclusive use of trained public health personnel, the brigades that inoculated the public relied heavily on "Servers of the Nation," political militants and volunteers that worked for social programmes that were closely associated with López Obrador's political party, MORENA. These 13-member brigades also included military personnel such that in total, they contained more social programme promoters and soldiers than medical and technical personnel (Sánchez Talanquer and Sepúlveda, 2024). There was absolutely no technical or medical justification for the involvement of the servers (Frenk and Gómez Dantés, 2021). Clearly, Operation Roadrunner had competing political/electoral and public health ends.

The government was also criticised for the politicised order of priority that it established to determine which segments of the population would be immunised first. Often against the recommendations of its own Technical Advisory Group for COVID-19 Vaccination (GTAV) and the WHO, it prioritised the application of vaccines to Servers of the Nation, doctors, and health workers who dealt with COVID-19 patients in public hospitals, teachers, and rural areas. With the exception of doctors and health workers in the public health sector, none of the others were considered priorities by GTAV. Notably, using a narrow definition of which health workers constituted priority targets, and despite their high risk of exposure to the virus, private doctors and healthcare workers were initially excluded from this priority list. It required a court order of the Supreme Court in May 2022 for health authorities to vaccinate these medical staff from private hospitals, clinics, and pharmacies, since they too formed part of the National Health System. Moreover, instead of privileging citizens with comorbidities for vaccination, authorities executed the roll-out by age groups (Frenk and Gómez Dantés, 2021; Sánchez Talanquer and Sepúlveda, 2024).

López-Gatell also drew heavy criticism for the delay in vaccinating youth and children. It took until June 2022 for the government to commence vaccinating children under 11 years of age, following legal action by worried parents. López-Gatell reasoned publicly, without scientific evidence, that children enjoyed more resilient immune systems against the virus, that it could even be harmful to immunise them, and hence it was more urgent to apply vaccines to higher-risk segments of the population (Díaz, 2022; García, 2023; Kane Jiménez and Gandy, 2021; Sánchez Talanquer and Sepúlveda, 2024, p. 272).

Finally, the government's choice of at least some vaccines to administer to the population was also politically motivated. Originally, during the first year of vaccination, with the urgent need to inoculate the population in the context of the failure of COVAX to provide adequate supply, the laudable efforts of the Secretariat of External Relations (SRE) to obtain vaccines were largely driven by pragmatism: to get the shots wherever they became available on short notice. This often meant playing the game of vaccine diplomacy with American, Chinese, Russian, and European donor governments. Accordingly, SRE arranged the purchase or donations of eight different vaccines: Abdalá, AstraZeneca, CanSino, Janssen, Moderna, Pfizer, Sinovac, and Sputnik V (Sánchez Talanquer and Sepúlveda, 2024).

Although they were not recommended by the WHO, Mexican authorities relied heavily on imports of the Russian vaccine Sputnik and the Cuban Abdalá, even when gradually a more plentiful supply of other authorised alternatives became available. Indeed, in December 2021, the Federal Commission for Protection against Health Risks (COFEPRIS) formally authorised the use of Abdalá, notwithstanding its lack of WHO or broader international approval or that the vaccine had solely undergone clinical trials in Cuba. Moreover, Mexican authorities decided to apply the vaccine to children, even though Pfizer was the only vaccine that possessed authorisation from the WHO for use in children under 5 years of age. Its Mexican adoption was underpinned by a formal bilateral agreement that López Obrador signed with his counterpart, Miguel Díaz-Canel, during an official visit to Cuba in May 2022, and for which the details of Mexico's vaccine purchase were not disclosed (Sotomayor, 2023). The application of both of these earlier generation vaccines was further questioned in 2022 and 2023 for whether they offered up-to-date protection against more recent strains of the coronavirus (Sánchez, 2023).

Lastly, the development of a homegrown vaccine, Patria, was also politically inspired. In the context of the urgent supply challenges of 2021, it did make a lot sense for the government to promote vaccine sovereignty, as López Obrador espoused publicly (Capital 21 Web, 2023; Universal, 2023). Even though the vaccine relied largely on technology developed in the United States by the Mount Sinai Icahn School of Medicine, it was politically packaged by López Obrador with a nationalistic name, Patria, inspired by the poem *Suave Patria* by Zacatecan Ramón López Velarde (Sánchez, 2023). In spite of the initial pledge of the government to have the vaccine approved and in production by the end of 2021 or early 2022, it took until January 2024 for Patria to complete its development, trials, and receive domestic authorisation by the Comité de Moléculas Nuevas (Committee for New Molecules) (AMLO, 2024) and June 2024 by COFEPRIS (Gobierno de México, 2024), long after Mexico and the WHO had officially declared an end to the COVID-19 public health emergency. Notwithstanding other technical and logistical challenges, the principal reason for Patria's slow development was the lack of adequate financing for the initiative (Sánchez, 2023), not surprising in the context of the government's *republican austerity*. Just as in the cases of Sputnik and Abdalá, critics questioned whether Patria's vaccine technology was out of date against more recent mutations of the COVID-19 virus (Flores, 2022; Sánchez, 2023).

Conclusion: Global Political Economy Meets Populism in Mexico's COVID-19 Vaccine Drive

In this chapter, I have argued that a pernicious combination of pandemic politics made its presence felt in the nexus between governance and government in Mexico's problematic COVID-19 vaccination experience. On one side, despite the widespread rhetoric among numerous international stakeholders about the paramountcy of vaccine equity and globalism and the need for pandemic vaccines to become a global public good, the global political economy proved fertile ground for the rise of a global pandemic vaccine governance complex that reflected the power of the countries and pharmaceutical companies that were concentrated largely in the Global North and favoured their interests. As I elaborated earlier, powerful global political economy tendencies distorted vaccine governance against greater equity and access by countries of the Global South in at least four important and interconnected ways: the design of governance institutions; the defence of intellectual property; vaccine nationalism and regionalism; and vaccine diplomacy. Although this governance complex fostered the fastest development of vaccines in human history, its vaccine arm, COVAX, failed to provide countries like Mexico with access to an adequate supply of vaccines for its population. Accordingly, Mexican authorities were left largely to defend themselves.

On the other side, the López Obrador government adopted a particular populist style of pandemic politics that weakened the country's vaccination performance considerably. Assorted and interconnected tendencies of what have been called medical populism, epistemological populism, presidential policy narrative, patrimonialism, and downsizing populism produced overarching centralisation and politicisation impulses that led to harmful consequences, for both the government's overall COVID-19 vaccination initiative and its statistics. The López Obrador vaccine strategy contributed to a successful effort to maintain the president's popularity rating and produce important electoral gains during the 2021 midterm elections (De la Cerda and Martínez-Gallardo, 2023), but it sacrificed the harnessing of a whole-of-government and whole-of-society approach.

Consequently, the country's vaccination process suffered important delays. Furthermore, certain groups who should have been among those prioritised were not, such as doctors and health workers who were not narrowly identified as directly on the COVID-19 frontline or who were from private hospitals, people with comorbidities, and children. Thanks in part to this politically motivated practice, Mexico suffered the highest mortality rate among physicians and health workers in the world (Dávila, 2023; Sánchez Talanquer and Sepúlveda, 2024, p. 278). On the basis of political criteria, authorities also opted to apply Russian and Cuban vaccines that were not recommended by the WHO and whose reliability against more recent strains of the virus has been questioned by experts.

Despite the government's pro-poor rhetoric, a two-tiered vaccine coverage evolved instead of vaccines as a truly public good. That is, whereas Mexico's lower-income groups have had to make do with public sector inoculations and booster shots that have often used inferior vaccines such as Sputnik, Abdalá, and soon Patria, more well-to-do Mexicans were able to resort to vaccine tourism to travel to the United States for more effective vaccines. Beginning in early 2024, a mixed public-private good regime prevailed, since Mexicans with adequate income could also now purchase more reputable booster shots like Pfizer from private pharmacies for the first time.

As Figures 4.1 and 4.2 highlighted, Mexico's overall vaccination rate was inferior to those of many other Latin American countries, as well as in comparison with the averages for high-income, upper-middle-income, South American, and North American countries. In all likelihood, thousands of Mexicans were unprotected, under-protected, or succumbed to COVID-19 unnecessarily, thanks to the pandemic politics of the country's vaccination experience. The lesson is clear: Until international stakeholders and Mexican authorities get the political economy and politics of global pandemic vaccine governance and public administration right, we can expect more of the same consequences in the event of future infectious disease outbreaks.

Notes

1 See also https://data.who.int/dashboards/covid19/vaccines?n=c.
2 Orchestration is a mode of governance in which intergovernmental organizations (IGO) "enlist intermediary actors on a voluntary basis, by providing them with ideational and material support, to address target actors in pursuit of IGO governance goals" (Abbott *et al.*, 2015, p. 3). On the WHO's role as a governance orchestrator, see Hanrieder (2015).
3 On governance gaps analysis, see Weiss (2013).
4 www.statista.com/statistics/1194813/latin-america-covid-19-vaccination-rate-country/.

References

Abbott, K.W. *et al.* (2015) 'Orchestration: global governance through intermediaries', in Abbott, K.W. *et al.* (eds.) *International organizations as orchestrators*. Cambridge: Cambridge University Press, pp. 3–36.

Alter, K.J. and Meunier, S. (2009) 'The politics of international regime complexity', *Perspectives on Politics*, 7(1), pp. 13–24.

Alter, K.J. and Raustiala, K. (2018) 'The rise of international regime complexity', *Annual Review of Law and Social Science*, 14(1), pp. 329–349.

AMLO (2024) 'Vacuna Patria es eficaz frente a variantes actuales de COVID-19; producción iniciará en febrero', *Official press site of Andrés Manuel López Obrador*, 30 January. Available at: https://lopezobrador.org.mx/2024/01/30/vacuna-patria-es-eficaz-frente-a-variantes-actuales-de-covid-19-produccion-iniciara-en-febrero/#:~:text=Adem%C3%A1s%2C%20ha%20mostrado%20efectividad%20equivalente,presidente%20Andr%C3%A9s%20Manuel%20L%C3%B3pez%20Obrador.

Bayerlein, M.V.A. *et al.* (2021) 'Populism and COVID-19: how populist governments (mis)handle the pandemic', *Journal of Political Institutions and Political Economy*, 2, pp. 389–428.

Biermann, F. *et al.* (2009) 'The fragmentation of global governance architectures: a framework for analysis', *Global Environmental Politics*, 9(4), pp. 14–40.

Bollyky, T.J. and Bown, C.P. (2020a) 'The tragedy of vaccine nationalism: only cooperation can end the pandemic', *Foreign Affairs*, 99(5), pp. 96–108.

Bollyky, T.J. and Bown, C.P. (2020b) 'Vaccine nationalism will prolong the pandemic: a global problem calls for collective action', *Foreign Affairs*, 29 December. Available at: www.foreignaffairs.com/articles/world/2020-12-29/vaccine-nationalism-will-prolong-pandemic.

Brende, B. *et al.* (2017) 'CEPI—a new global R&D organization for epidemic preparedness and response', *The Lancet*, 389(10066), pp. 233–235.

Brubaker, R. (2017) 'Why populism?', *Theory and Society*, 46, pp. 357–385.

Capital 21 Web. (2023) '¡Tenemos "Patria"! Vacuna contra COVID-19 de México está lista', *Capital 21 Web*. Available at: www.capital21.cdmx.gob.mx/noticias/?p=30479.

Commission on Global Governance (1995) *Our global neighborhood: the report of the commission on global governance*. Oxford, UK: Oxford University Press.

Dávila, P. (2023) 'COVID-19: Los pecados de López Gatell que la Fiscalía debe investigar', *Proceso*, June 10. Available at: https://www.proceso.com.mx/reportajes/2023/6/10/covid-19-los-pecados-de-lopez-gatell-que-la-fiscalia-debe-investigar-308589.html.

de Bengy Puyvallée, A. (2024) 'The rising authority and agency of public—private partnerships in global health governance', *Policy and Society*, 43(1), pp. 25–40.

de Bengy Puyvallée, A. and Storeng, K.T. (2022) 'COVAX, vaccine donations and the politics of global vaccine inequity', *Global Health*, 18(26), pp. 1–14.

De la Cerda, N. and Martínez-Gallardo, C. (2023) 'Mexico: a politically effective populist pandemic response', in Ringe, N. and Renno, L. (eds.) *Populists and the pandemic: how populists around the world responded to COVID-19*. New York and London: Routledge, pp. 29–43.

Díaz, P. (2022) 'Gobierno no adquirió suficientes vacunas contra la influenza: Francisco Moreno', *Excélsior*, 12 December. Available at: www.excelsior.com.mx/nacional/autoridades-sanitarias-han-descuidado-vacunacion/1558697.

Dresser, D. (2022) 'Mexico's dying democracy: AMLO and the toll of authoritarian populism', *Foreign Affairs*, November–December. Available at: www.foreignaffairs.com/mexico/mexico-dying-democracy-amlo-toll-authoritarian-populism-denise-dresser.

Dresser, D. (2024) 'Mexico's vote for autocracy: how AMLO undermined democracy and brought back party dominance', *Foreign Affairs, Snapshot*, 17 May. Available at: www.foreignaffairs.com/mexico/mexicos-vote-autocracy.

Dussauge-Laguna, M.I. (2022) 'The promises and perils of populism for democratic policymaking: the case of Mexico', *Policy Sciences*, 55, pp. 777–803.

Eilstrup-Sangiovanni, M. and Westerwinter, O. (2022) 'The global governance complexity cube: varieties of institutional complexity in global governance', *Review of International Organizations*, 17, pp. 233–262.

Flores, J. (2022) 'Vacuna "Patria": tardía e ineficaz', *Grupo Milenio*. Available at: www.milenio.com/nexos/vacuna-patria-tardia-e-ineficaz (Accessed 7 June 2024).

Frenk, J. and Gómez Dantés, O. (2021) 'Opinión: 'Patria' o ciencia: contradicciones de la vacuna mexicana contra COVID-19', *Washington Post*, 19 April. Available at: www.washingtonpost.com/es/post-opinion/2021/04/19/vacuna-patria-mexicana-covid-19-amlo/.

García, I. (2023) 'A tres años de la pandemia de Covid siguen las críticas a Gatell', *Azteca Noticias*. Available at: www.tvazteca.com/aztecanoticias/a-tres-anos-de-la-pandemia-de-covid-siguen-las-criticas-a-gatell-cs (Accessed 28 May 2024).

Geiger, S. and McMahon, A. (2021) 'Analysis of the institutional landscape and proliferation of proposals for global vaccine equity for COVID-19: too many cooks or too many recipes?', *Journal of Medical Ethics*, 49(8), pp. 583–590.

Georgieva, K. *et al.* (2021) *A new commitment for vaccine equity and defeating the pandemic.* World Health Organization. Available at: www.who.int/news-room/commentaries/detail/a-new-commitment-for-vaccine-equity-and-defeating-the-pandemic.

Gobierno de México (2024, 6 June) *Cofepris aprueba la vacuna mexicana Patria contra COVID-19.* Comisión Federal para la Protección contra Riesgos Sanitarios, Comunicado 79/2024. Available at: www.gob.mx/cofepris/articulos/cofepris-aprueba-la-vacuna-mexicana-patria-contra-covid-19#:~:text=El%20equipo%20multidisciplinario%20de%20dictamen,las%20instituciones%20p%C3%BAbli cas%20que%20conforman.

Gouglas, D. *et al.* (2019) 'CEPI: driving progress toward epidemic preparedness and response', *Epidemiologic Reviews*, 41(1), pp. 28–33.

Gratius, S., Legler, T. and Quezada, J. (2021) 'La Gobernanza Regional Del Covid-19 en La Unión Europea Y América Latina Y El Caribe', *Anuario de la Facultad de Derecho de la Universidad Autónoma de Madrid*, 25, pp. 59–92. Available at: https://search.ebscohost.com/login.aspx?direct=true&AuthType=ip,url,uid&db=fa p&AN=157786438&lang=es&site=eds-live&scope=sit.

Guilbaud, A. (2023) 'A stress-test for global health multilateralism: the COVID-19 pandemic as revealer and catalyst of cooperation challenges', in Guilbaud, A., Petiteville, F. and Ramel, F. (eds.) *Crisis of multilateralism? Challenges and resilience.* Cham, CH: Palgrave Macmillan, pp. 47–76.

Hanrieder, T. (2015) 'WHO orchestrates? Coping with competitors in global health', in Abbott, K.W. *et al.* (eds.) *International organizations as orchestrators.* Cambridge, UK: Cambridge University Press, pp. 191–213.

Hanson, S. and Kopstein, J. (2021) 'Understanding the global patrimonial wave', *Perspectives on Politics*, 20(1), pp. 237–249.

Huneycutt, B. *et al.* (2020) 'Finding equipoise: CEPI revises its equitable access policy', *Vaccine*, 38(9), pp. 2144–2148.

Infobae (2021) 'Nuestro único gran proyecto debe ser salvar vidas: Krauze y Aguilar Camín piden a AMLO detener megaproyectos y cambiar estrategia contra el COVID-19', *Infobae*, February 9. Available at: https://www.infobae.com/america/mexico/2021/02/09/nuestro-unico-gran-proyecto-debe-ser-salvar-vidas-krauze-y-aguilar-camin-piden-a-amlo-detener-megaproyectos-y-cambiar-estrategia-contra-el-covid-19/.

KaneJiménez, S. and Gandy, A. (2021, 4 October) *Infographic: Mexico's vaccine supply and distribution efforts.* Wilson Center. Available at: www.wilsoncenter.org/article/infographic-mexicos-vaccine-supply-and-distribution-efforts.

Kieny, M.P. and Salama, P. (2017) 'WHO R&D blueprint: a global coordination mechanism for R&D preparedness', *The Lancet*, 389(10088), pp. 2469–2470.

King Mantilla, K. and Carranza Barona, C. (2022) *COVID-19 vaccines as global public goods: between life and profit.* Geneva: South Centre, p. 154. Available at: https://hdl.handle.net/10419/262129.

Krishnan, V. (2021) 'How to end vaccine apartheid', *Foreign Policy*, 9 November. Available at: https://foreignpolicy.com/2021/11/09/vaccine-apartheid-covid-pandemic-covax-us-trips-waiver/.

Lasco, G. (2020) 'Medical populism and the COVID-19 pandemic', *Global Public Health*, 15(10), pp. 1417–1429.

Lasco, G. and Curato, N. (2019) 'Medical populism', *Social Science & Medicine*, 221, pp. 1–8.

Lurie, N., Keusch, G.T. and Dzau, V.J. (2021) 'Urgent lessons from COVID 19: why the world needs a standing, coordinated system and sustainable financing for global research and development', *The Lancet*, 397(10280), pp. 1229–1236.

Malacalza, B., and Fagaburu, D. (2022) '¿Empatía o cálculo? Un análisis crítico de la geopolítica de las vacunas en América Latina', *Foro Internacional*, 62(1), pp. 5–45.

Matthiessen, L. *et al.* (2016) 'Coordinating funding in public health emergencies', *The Lancet*, 387(10034), pp. 2197–2198.

McNeill, D. and Sandberg, K. (2014) 'Trust in global health governance: the GAVI experience', *Global Governance*, 20(2), pp. 325–343.

Moreno, P. (2022) *Historias de una pandemia: El relato del infectólogo de referencia sobre el coronavirus y sus impesansables consecuencias.* Mexico City: Penguin Random House.

Natal, A. (2021) 'For the sake of all, the poor first: COVID-19, mañaneras, and the popularity of the Mexican president', in Fernandez, M. and Machado, C. (eds.) *COVID-19's political challenges in Latin America.* Cham, CH: Springer, pp. 163–181.

Orsini, A., Morin, J.-F. and Young, O. (2013) 'Regime complexes: a buzz, a boom, or a boost for global governance?', *Global Governance*, 19(1), pp. 27–39.

Peci, A., González, C. and Dussauge-Laguna, M.I. (2022) 'Presidential policy narratives and the (mis)use of scientific expertise: COVID-19 policy responses in Brazil, Colombia, and Mexico', *Policy Studies*, 44(1), pp. 68–89.

Raustiala, K. and Victor, D.G. (2004) 'The regime complex for plant genetic resources', *International Organization*, 58(2), pp. 277–309.

Redacción. (2023) 'Vacunas Abdala y Sputnik "no son útiles" vs. el COVID, afirma Francisco Moreno', *El Financiero*, 23 October. Available at: www.elfinanciero.com.mx/nacional/2023/10/23/vacunas-abdala-y-sputnik-no-son-utiles-afirma-el-dr-francisco-moreno.

Renteria, C. and Arellano-Gault, D. (2021) 'How does a populist government interpret and face a health crisis? Evidence from the Mexican populist response to COVID-19', *Revista de Administração Pública*, 55(1), pp. 180–196.

Reuters (2021) 'A year in the COVID-19 vaccine scheme COVAX', *Reuters*, 21 April. Available at: www.reuters.com/business/healthcare-pharmaceuticals/year-covid-19-vaccine-scheme-covax-2021-04-21/.

Sánchez, I. (2023) 'Patria: a la espera de la vacuna prometida', *Reforma*, 15 October. Available at: www.reforma.com/patria-a-la-espera-de-la-vacuna-prometida/ar2687110.

Sánchez Talanquer, M. and Sepúlveda, J. (eds.) (2024) *Informe de la Comisión Independiente de Investigación sobre la Pandemia de Covid-19 en México.* Mexico City. Available at: www.comisioncovid.mx/.

Sánchez-Talanquer, M. *et al.* (2021) *Mexico's response to COVID-19: a case study.* San Francisco: Institute for Global Health Sciences, University of California, San Francisco. Available at: https://globalhealthsciences.ucsf.edu/wp-content/uploads/2024/02/mexico-covid-19-case-study-english.pdf.

Sandberg, K.I., Andresen, S. and Bjune, G. (2010) 'A new approach to global health institutions? A case study of new vaccine introduction and the formation of the GAVI Alliance', *Social Science & Medicine*, 71(7), pp. 1349–1356.

Saurette, P. and Gunster, S. (2011) 'Ears wide shut: epistemological populism, argutainment and Canadian conservative talk radio', *Canadian Journal of Political Science*, 44(1), pp. 195–218.

Shu, Y. and McCauley, J. (2017) 'GISAID: global initiative on sharing all influenza data—from vision to reality', *Euro Surveillance*, 22(13), pp. 1–3.

Sotomayor, G. (2023) 'Abdala, la vacuna de Cuba que se aplica en México, aún carece de aval de la OMS', *Proceso*, May 9. Available at: https://www.proceso.com.mx/nacional/2023/5/9/abdala-la-vacuna-de-cuba-que-se-aplica-en-mexico-aun-carece-de-aval-de-la-oms-306715.html.

Storeng, K.T., de Bengy Puyvallée, A. and Stein, F. (2023) 'COVAX and the rise of the "super public private partnership" for global health', *Global Public Health*, 18(1), pp. 1–17.

Theil, S. (2021) 'The year vaccines changed (most) of the world', *Foreign Policy*, 22 December. Available at: https://foreignpolicy.com/2021/12/22/2021-vaccines-covid-pandemic/.

Touchton, M. *et al.* (2023) 'The perilous mix of populism and pandemics: lessons from COVID-19', *Social Sciences*, 12(7), pp. 1–9.

United Nations General Assembly (2020a) 'Global solidarity to fight the coronavirus disease 2019 (COVID-19)', *Resolution 74/270*, 2 April. Available at: https://documents.un.org/doc/undoc/gen/n20/087/28/pdf/n2008728.pdf?token=ODQJs81y0QllVTe7RV&fe=true.

United Nations General Assembly (2020b) 'International cooperation to ensure global access to medicines, vaccines and medical equipment to face COVID-19', *Resolution 74/274*, 20 April. Available at: https://documents.un.org/doc/undoc/gen/n20/101/42/pdf/n2010142.pdf?token=XHOZXNJL6r7CbmBJqS&fe=true.

Universal (2023) 'Vacuna se llama "Patria" para recordar a los mexicanos sobre soberanía nacional e independencia: AMLO', *El Universal*, 13 April. Available at: https://www.eluniversal.com.mx/nacion/amlo-vacuna-se-llama-patria-para-recordar-los-mexicanos-sobre-soberania-nacional-e/.

Valderrama, B. *et al.* (2021) 'Vaccine diplomacy and political diversification in Mexico's science and technology stakeholders', *Science & Diplomacy*, 6 February. Available at: www.sciencediplomacy.org/article/2021/vaccine-diplomacy-and-political-diversification-in-mexicos-science-and-technology.

Venkatesan, P. (2023, 13 October) 'New licences for the COVID-19 technology access pool', *The Lancet Microbe*, 4(12).

Weiss, T.G. (2013) *Global governance: why? what? whither?* Cambridge, UK: Polity Press.

World Health Assembly (2020) 'COVID-19 response', *Resolution WHA73.1*, 19 May. Available at: https://apps.who.int/gb/ebwha/pdf_files/WHA73/A73_R1-en.pdf.

World Health Organization (2005) *International health regulations*. Geneva: World Health Organization. Available at: https://iris.who.int/bitstream/handle/10665/246107/9789241580496-eng.pdf?sequence=1.

World Health Organization (2006) *Global pandemic influenza action plan to increase vaccine supply*, Geneva: World Health Organization. Available at: www.who.int/publications/i/item/WHO-CDS-EPR-GIP-2006-1.

World Health Organization (2011) *Pandemic influenza preparedness framework*. Geneva: World Health Organization. Available at: pandemic-influenza-preparedness-en.pdf (who.int).

World Health Organization (2012) *Report of the WHO pandemic influenza A(H1N1) vaccine deployment initiative*. Geneva: World Health Organization. Available at: https://iris.who.int/bitstream/handle/10665/44795/9789241564427_eng.pdf?sequence=1.

World Health Organization (2019) *Global influenza strategy 2019–2030*. Geneva: World Health Organization. Available at: https://iris.who.int/bitstream/handle/10665/311184/9789241515320-eng.pdf?sequence=18

World Health Organization (2021) *Strategy to achieve global Covid-19 vaccination by mid-2022*. Available at: https://cdn.who.int/media/docs/default-source/immunization/covid-19/strategy-to-achieve-global-covid-19-vaccination-by-mid-2022.pdf?sfvrsn=5a68433c_5&download=true.

World Health Organization (2023) 'Increasing COVID-19 vaccination uptake: an update on messaging, delivery strategies and policy recommendations', *Information Note*, December. Available at: https://cdn.who.int/media/docs/default-source/agenda-sage/information-note---increasing-covid-19-vaccination.pdf?sfvrsn=6ce03e0c_2&download=true.

Ximénez Fyvie, L.A. (2021) *Un daño irreparable: La criminal gestión de la pandemia en México*. Mexico City: Editorial Planeta.

Ximénez Fyvie, L.A. (2022) *Las vidas que no contaron*. Mexico City: Editorial Planeta.

Yadav, P. (2021) 'How to make COVID-19 vaccines available to all: manufacture the right kinds in the right places', *Foreign Affairs, Snapshot*, 27 December. Available at: www.foreignaffairs.com/articles/world/2021-12-27/how-make-covid-19-vaccines-available-all.

Yamey, G. *et al.* (2022, 24 March) 'It is not too late to achieve global covid-19 vaccine equity', *British Medical Journal*, 376, p. e070650. Available at: www.bmj.com/content/bmj/376/bmj-2022-070650.full.pdf.

5 Multistakeholder Partnerships for Migrant Healthcare Access at the US-Mexico Border (San Diego-Tijuana) During the COVID-19 Pandemic

Valeria Marina Valle, Caroline Irene Deschak and Michelle Ruiz Valdes[1]

Introduction

In 2015, the United Nations (UN) member states unanimously committed to implementing the 17 Sustainable Development Goals (SDGs) by the year 2030. A variety of actions have been implemented in an effort to achieve these goals. Nevertheless, the COVID-19 pandemic and its societal repercussions brought unprecedented socio-political challenges with consequences for all the goals, particularly SDGs 3 (health), 10 (equality), and 17 (partnerships).

The objective of this chapter is to conduct a comprehensive analysis of cooperation dynamics between different stakeholders mandated with facilitating access to COVID-19-related healthcare and vaccination for migrants along the US-Mexico border, specifically in the San Diego-Tijuana region, during the early stages of the COVID-19 pandemic (2020–2021). Through the lens of disease diplomacy, we aim to understand how these partnerships functioned under the pressures of the pandemic, what strategies were implemented to overcome barriers to healthcare rights for migrants, and the effectiveness of these efforts against SDGs 3, 10, and 17. We ask: How did actors on both sides of the border interact during the pandemic to ensure or impede the provision of healthcare services to migrants?

Disease diplomacy is the collaborative effort among states and international actors to enhance disease surveillance and control. It involves the collective endeavour to achieve global health security by adhering to the revised 2005 International Health Regulations, which aim to address challenges in disease control and promote cooperation among nations for safeguarding global health (Davies, Kamradt-Scott, and Rushton, 2015). Disease diplomacy is a form of international cooperation crucial to managing and controlling the spread of diseases, particularly in border zones where human movement can exacerbate the transmission of infectious disease. By understanding the collaborative efforts of border actors, including multi-level (local, regional, national, international) and multi-sectoral (state, non-state) actors, we can assess the effectiveness of public health strategies during a pandemic.

Through its emphasis on multilevel governance (MLG), disease diplomacy is instrumental to achieving the SDGs, especially those aimed at ensuring that health and well-being are rights for all, regardless of age, origin, nationality, and gender. This underscores the relevance of disease diplomacy in promoting equitable global health, in line with goals set at both the international and local levels.

This chapter focuses on San Diego (United States) and Tijuana (Mexico), which together form the most-crossed international border in the Western world. Tijuana in particular is considered a key transit area on the migratory route, known as the "city without borders" (IOM, 2015, p. 49) as a nod to the complex and constant mobility of people. However, according to the *World Migration Report 2015*, this quality appears weakened due to the political measures by the United States and Mexico that interrupt mobility and contain migrants who must wait for the right opportunity to move.

To analyse the interactions between actors in the border region, we used a combined methodology for data collection: (1) primary qualitative data through electronic written questionnaires to key informants and (2) secondary data through scientific and grey literature (news sources, reports from governmental and non-governmental programmes). Fifteen questionnaires were answered by active contributors from academic, civil society, or public sector organisations, each with between three and 22 years (average: ten) of experience in the migration field. Most lived and worked in Tijuana and brought perspectives from the Mexican side of the border.

Most participants (eight) held key positions within civil society organisations (CSOs) in Mexico providing direct services to the migrant population. These included directors, general and medical coordinators, attorneys, and regional representatives, some of whom collaborated closely with colleagues on both sides of the border. Of these, several were medical doctors. At least two participants who principally worked within CSOs were also involved in higher academic institutions in Tijuana. Most CSOs represented by participants specifically served the migrant or refugee population (Centro 32/ Families Belong Together Mexico, Espacio Migrante A.C., Desayunador/ Albergue Salesiano Padre Chava, Refugee Health Alliance (RHA), Al Otro Lado), although two also served wider audiences in need of diverse social support (Prevencasa, American Friends Service Committee—Latin America and Caribbean). One informant came from an international organisation: the United Nations International Organization for Migration (IOM).

Five participants identified as professors or researchers with a focus on migration topics. Their affiliated academic institutions were mainly Mexican (Universidad Nacional Autónoma de México, Universidad Iberoamericana Mexico City, El Colegio de la Frontera Norte), with one in the United States (University of California at Davis). Finally, one actor was employed in the

Mexican public sector, playing a coordination role in the General Consulate of Mexico in San Diego. Information from the questionnaires is presented with the express informed consent of the actors.

The chapter is divided into two sections. The first presents disease diplomacy in the context of the COVID-19 pandemic, emphasising its increasing importance as a framework for navigating a complex global health landscape. The second section presents dynamics and challenges in providing healthcare services for migrants in the San Diego-Tijuana border region during the pandemic.

Disease Diplomacy as Analytical Framework: Links With MLG and the 2030 Agenda

Disease diplomacy takes on an amplified significance in the context of the COVID-19 pandemic as a framework for navigating an evolving global health landscape. The pandemic has starkly demonstrated that international actors (from states to NGOs) often face challenges in synchronising responses due to diverse political agendas, resource constraints, and differing capacities.

Disease diplomacy has become especially prominent in the literature on pandemic politics, where the need for a unified and effective response has highlighted the importance of diplomatic strategies that can manage public health within the MLG framework and in alignment with the 2030 Agenda. Thus, disease diplomacy seeks not only to contain disease outbreaks but also to strengthen health systems in the long term and promote equity in health access.

This approach is based on the premise that actors from different sectors (state, intergovernmental, and non-state) interact at multiple levels with respect to disease surveillance and control (Davies *et al.*, 2015). These interactions can be classified into three distinct types of diplomacy: core or formal diplomacy; multistakeholder diplomacy; and informal diplomacy (Katz *et al.*, 2011; see also Ruckert *et al.*, 2016). Core or formal diplomacy, involving high-level political negotiations and agreements between states, is essential for formulating global health policies and frameworks that align with the SDGs. This type of diplomacy can lead to the establishment of international norms and commitments, such as those aimed at ending epidemics and ensuring healthy lives for all (SDGs 3 and 10).

Multistakeholder diplomacy brings together a diverse range of actors beyond nation-states, including NGOs, private sector players, and international organisations. This type of diplomacy is aligned with SDG 17, which emphasises partnerships to reach the goals. Through collaboration, these various stakeholders can pool resources, expertise, and implementation capacities vital to achieving the comprehensive and inclusive approach to health envisioned in the 2030 Agenda.

Informal diplomacy operates outside official diplomatic channels and often involves civil society, academic institutions, and health professionals.

These actors can influence policy through advocacy, create awareness, and drive community-level action, which is fundamental for the localisation of the SDGs. Informal diplomacy supports the MLG framework by facilitating the flow of information and best practices across different governance levels, from local to global, ensuring that initiatives are responsive to community needs and grounded in local realities.

Although there is no consensus around the definition of MLG, this approach has been a *leitmotif* of integration processes in European studies (Castro-Conde, 2010). Its reach has extended to other areas in environmental and social issues, such as migration (Libert-Amico *et al.*, 2018; Ortega, 2021). In this chapter, MLG is defined as "the dispersion of authority outside the central government, upwards to the supranational level, downwards to subnational jurisdictions, and laterally to public-private networks" (Hooghe and Marks, 2002, 2003, cited in Panizzon and van Riemsdijk, 2019, p. 1226). On the basis of a review of the literature on governance, this dispersion is considered to have the objective of providing goods and services (Risse, 2011).

The original concept of MLG, proposed by Hooghe and Marks (2002), included a Type I and Type II governance scheme (Panizzon and van Riemsdijk, 2019). Type I refers to a limited number of jurisdictions (international, national, regional, meso, local) with a general purpose, clear boundaries, and permanent configuration, which focuses power and decision-making on a limited number of actors (mainly governments). In contrast, Type II consists of flexible and ambiguous jurisdictions characterised by their overlap and interconnection. Type II schemes are readily identifiable in border regions, where functional jurisdictions are composed of multiple state or non-state actors operating to solve problems and provide services (Castro-Conde, 2010; Panizzon and van Riemsdijk, 2019).

As mentioned, MLG has expanded to issues such as migration (Panizzon and van Riemsdijk, 2019; Scholten and Penninx, 2016), where distinct classifications have been proposed as shown in Table 5.1.

Notably, throughout this classification scheme, one variable analysed is the interaction between actors at jurisdictional or territorial levels. Sometimes these are orchestrated, with policies adopted and implemented across levels, but at other times they are disjointed, as in the case of the decoupled mode. This may be not only due to divergent interests but also due to the way in which each actor involved may define a problem or neglect to share information with others (Porras, 2021). The localist mode focused on bottom-up processes recognises that at the local level there are problems that need to be addressed by the actors who experience them or have local legitimacy. The MLG model shows clear links to disease diplomacy since the latter allows analysis of the performance of government actors and the role of other actors in crisis management. Transgovernmental networks are found within a multi-actor and multilevel reality.

Table 5.1 Classification and main characteristics of multilevel governance in the context of migration

Classification	Main characteristics
Centralist mode	Top-down relations that exhibit a clear hierarchy, division of labour, and control mechanisms between government levels to ensure policy implementation through a vertical coherence approach
Localist mode	Bottom-up perspective where political implementing bodies or regional actors follow the principle that "what can be done locally must be done locally" (Scholten and Penninx, 2016, p. 93)
Multilevel style	Interactions and joint coordination-style relations without a clear hierarchical dominance, exercised through forums or networks in which organisations of different mandates are involved in a specific policy domain
Decoupled mode	The absence of meaningful interactions at multiple levels

Source: Created by the authors, based on Scholten (2013) and Scholten and Penninx (2016)

"Disengagement" (decoupled mode) in the migratory field results in national authorities distancing themselves from local phenomena and therefore holding others accountable for their management, including migrants themselves (Ortega, 2021). Faced with decoupling, horizontal networks have been created, which invoke the capacities and interests of multiple stakeholders (Panizzon and van Riemsdijk, 2019).

Migration scholars such as Müller (2014) have highlighted that in border microregions, such as San Diego-Tijuana-Mexicali, local actors can act through networks to obtain resources (both in-kind and financial) and strengthen their capacity to negotiate with public officials. This demonstrates the heterogeneity of networks.

According to Müller, although transnational movements exist at the binational level, in the region of interest it is more relevant to consider cross-border networks. This is because, although the state has an important role in relations, lasting connections are present in the local civil society sector (Müller, 2014). Under this cross-border approach, it can be said that governance is local, whereby regional actors are guided by the principle that "what can be done locally must be done locally" (Scholten and Penninx, 2016, p. 93). Notably, this type of governance does not contradict the multilevel style since local actors come into contact with other national and binational non-governmental actors to obtain different resources.

A focus on healthcare services allows the identification of actors charged with addressing health within a region or where these actors have influence (Barragán, Riaño and Martínez, 2012; Quiroga, 2019). These services may be first, second, or third level (Barragán, Riaño and Martínez, 2012). The World Health Organization (WHO) has declared the provision of healthcare services and production of vaccines and medicines key to avoiding health risks. In vaccine and medicine production, the relationship between the government and private sector requires particular focus to ensure access to necessary goods. Therefore, the WHO recognises that ensuring access to these products depends on governance, information, human resources, and partnerships or relationships between multiple stakeholders in a given territory (WHO, 2018).

From this territorial standpoint, the 2030 Agenda advocates for a multilevel approach to encompass regional, national, and subnational levels through planning, capacity building, institutional development, and evaluation. Moreover, it involves initiatives driven by the private sector and other non-state stakeholders. This convergence of actors aligns with the concept of multistakeholder partnerships MSPs, and within the scope of disease diplomacy, it particularly resonates with the practices of multistakeholder diplomacy.

Considering the above, the following section analyses the types of interactions among a diversity of actors during the 2020–2021 period of the COVID-19 pandemic in the Tijuana-San Diego border region.

Migrant Healthcare Access in a Global Health Crisis: Actors and Interactions to "Leave No One Behind" in the Tijuana-San Diego Region During the COVID-19 Pandemic (2020–2021)

Healthcare services, far from being strictly a state function, are theoretically available to migrants through a patchwork of multisectoral actors and sustained by the partnerships among them. Around Tijuana, pandemic-era services were principally provided to migrant people by civil society and non-governmental organisations, followed by private pharmacies, and only distantly followed by public sector services.

A network of CSOs active in Mexico offers integrated services for health and wellness to the migrant community. Key among those who offer direct medical services, as mentioned by various informants, are the RHA and affiliates, Prevencasa, Centro 32, and Pro-Salud. Volunteer-based clinics within humanitarian spaces such as the Desayunador Padre Chava (Proyecto Salesiano) were also an important part of the network, even providing specialised services to address the needs of particularly vulnerable groups like the Midwifery and Ancestral Medicine Center (RHA).

The interactions described, involving collaborations and partnerships beyond the constraints of governmental or intergovernmental policies, align closely with the concept of informal disease diplomacy. They represent relationships outside the realm of formal diplomacy, specifically aimed at fostering action at the community level. This approach exemplifies the essence of informal disease diplomacy, which thrives on grassroots initiatives and cross-sectoral cooperation, bypassing the often slower and more rigid structures of formal diplomacy.

The Mexican Red Cross was an available option for emergency transport and care, but the high cost of services was prohibitive for most migrants. Networks between local CSOs in related sectors fomented community access and comprehensive services. These were, for example, links to churches, LGBTQ+ support organisations, and politically liberal organisations characterised by informants as being structured upon US models.

The latter is not a coincidence since binational collaborations for migration issues between organisations in the United States and Mexico have been present since long before the pandemic. According to Agudo (2020),

> [T]he initiatives and alliances between different centres and organisations that work with the Lesbian, Gay, Bisexual, Transgender, and Intersex population in Baja California are an example of the organisational effervescence and proliferation of non-governmental associations in the current context of border reinforcement, discrimination and criminalization of different populations produced by the current migration control policies.
>
> (Agudo, 2020, p. 65)

Despite clear economic and social advantages to CSO service provision, important capacity gaps were highlighted as a consistent concern. As a CSO director in Mexico emphasised,

> Few organisations directly provide healthcare services . . . we know that not everyone from the population in the context of mobility can access these services through organisations; that's why partnerships are created to link people in the migration context to different public and/ or private healthcare institutions.

This underscores the need for collaborative efforts to bridge the gap in healthcare access and highlights the essential role of partnerships in enhancing the reach and effectiveness of healthcare services provided by CSOs.

Therefore, another key role of civil society actors was maintaining strong connections with other multisectoral actors to support medical referral and, significantly, even physical accompaniment to public sector services. These were key actions of non-governmental actors at the local, national, binational, and international levels. MLG is evident in these types of interactions and joint coordination relationships, where diverse types of organisations are involved in a specific policy domain. The findings presented here suggest the need to consider an additional MLG classification focused on multi-sectoral relationships.

This multi-sectoral model appears aligned with methodological guidelines by the Economic Commission for Latin America and the Caribbean (ECLAC) for the planning of the 2030 Agenda, which "underlines the inadequate way of approaching complex sustainability problems, with the traditional perspective in the formulation of policies and planning, from thematic silos by specific sectors" (ECLAC, 2018, p. 13). The networks described in the Tijuana-San Diego migration context exemplify the cross-sector and cross-border collaborations characteristic of multistakeholder diplomacy.

Informants also acknowledged the frequent use of private medical services among migrants. While the high cost of private clinics often precluded their use, many were reported to prefer the abundant range of large-chain private pharmacies in Mexico. These pharmacies generally offered relatively afford-able and sometimes free medical consultations in addition to prescription drugs. However, these services are market-driven, oriented towards pharma-ceutical treatments, not necessarily compliant with epidemiological report-ing, and without continuous and comprehensive service options.

Evidently, least preferred by the migrant population were public sector health services managed by the Health Secretariat of Baja California, includ-ing clinics, health centres, and hospitals. In public sector installations, dis-crimination towards migrants was frequently described, even for Mexican nationals from other states and international migrants with regular status. Those who successfully received services were nearly always escorted by members of CSOs with established networks. Informants also mentioned the relatively new Integrative Migrant Centres (*Centros integradores para el migrante*), though their role was not seen as central within the network of public sector services. Additionally, the IMSS-Wellness Program (*Programa IMSS-Bienestar*) in 2020 provided consultations to migrants through seven service points in Mexican territory, including the "Carmen Serdán" Integra-tive Migrant Centre in Tijuana. The IMSS-Wellness Program had primary, secondary, and tertiary infrastructure in order to focus on vaccination and epidemiological surveillance. However, this centre was not seen as a viable option for many migrants who stay in shelters or in *El Chaparral* encamp-ments on the Mexican side of one official border crossing, and those who lack reliable and safe transportation. The centre was constructed at a dis-tance from *El Chaparral* and the international border with the United States (Ramírez, 2021).

This situation underscores the crucial role of NGOs in bridging the gap between the migrant community and the public healthcare sector. As noted by a researcher informant in Mexico,

> [I]n cases where better or more integral medical attention is needed, the NGOs are the ones who contact and refer migrant individuals to public hospitals. This is done to prevent institutional abuse in medical services (at least upon first entry).

The NGOs' involvement, therefore, becomes pivotal in ensuring that migrants can safely and effectively navigate the public system. This dynamic highlights a complex healthcare landscape where the collaboration between

CSOs and public health institutions is essential yet fraught with challenges and dependencies.

The above further demonstrates that in the provision of healthcare services to migrants, informal disease diplomacy through NGOs is key to avoiding institutional abuses and addressing the specific needs of migrants at the community level. Likewise, the work of these actors is linked to the localist model of MLG, as they demonstrate a territorial approach in identifying and addressing needs.

The IOM has noted that during the pandemic three types of administrative and systemic barriers influenced the experiences of migrants in vaccine access: low, medium, and high level. Low-level measures refer to any form of identification—valid or not, expired or not, and from anywhere—to verify identity. Medium level refers to certified documents (e.g., residence permit, host country insurance cards), though these may be accepted even if they have expired. High measures require specific types of documents that are still valid/unexpired (IOM, 2021).

In light of the situation in Mexico, it is evident that systemic measures for COVID-19 vaccine distribution and access were rated between medium and high in terms of their effectiveness and reach. However, practical challenges remained significant. As a medical doctor and co-director of a CSO in Mexico highlighted,

> [T]he COVID-19 vaccines, though available to adults based on age groups, are administered in locations that are often quite distant and expensive to travel to. Furthermore, without a CURP (Unique Population Registry Code), obtaining vaccination certification becomes an impossibility, even after receiving the vaccine.

This underscores the logistical and bureaucratic hurdles faced, particularly by those in marginalised groups, in accessing essential healthcare services like vaccination.

No sustained public sector mechanisms were identified that sought to guarantee migrant access to the COVID-19 vaccine. In fact, one informant expressed that migrants were only vaccinated in moments of surplus, and another mentioned that vaccination was strictly discretionary because the only way to get access was through direct accompaniment by a figure with network influence. While the health jurisdiction was seen to have made sporadic efforts to address COVID-19 in other aspects, no concerted effort was recognised, and while some shelters managed to hold their own vaccination campaigns, these were only possible with support to obtain the highly coveted vaccines.

As one sub-director of a CSO in Mexico noted, *"in some shelters, there is access to COVID-19 vaccines through organisations from the United States. The majority of the population still doesn't have open access; migrants are only offered vaccines when there is an excess of supply."* Selective and intermittent vaccine provision underscores the broader challenges of COVID-19 vaccine availability for the general public in Mexico, especially during the early phases of global vaccine distribution.

This sporadic targeted provision of vaccines was nonetheless important, particularly given the scarcity of vaccine supply available to the general public in Mexico, even more evident at the beginning stages of global vaccine distribution. Global attention to the pandemic also fostered opportunities for CSOs to receive resources to specifically dedicate to combating COVID-19.

As a Programme Officer from a CSO in Mexico noted,

[T]here are no specific campaigns targeting migrant individuals for vaccine access. In Tijuana, some shelters organised vaccination campaigns, but this was not widespread. The health jurisdiction of the Health Ministry occasionally conducted workshops and offered COVID-19 tests and information on isolation procedures in shelters, but not all shelters received such assistance. In fact, some shelters that formally requested help did not receive any response.

This statement highlights the patchy and often inadequate response of the public health system, underscoring a pressing need for more structured and consistent support, especially in obtaining highly sought-after vaccines for vulnerable shelter populations.

Federal law in Mexico allows open access to COVID-19 vaccines for all eligible individuals, independent of his or her migratory status. In theory, this allowed unfettered vaccine access to migrants. This happened in some places, such as one participant, for example, who affirmed that although help arrived late, migrant shelters, assistance points, and even the migrant encampment at *El Chaparral* did receive some vaccines. Moreover, periodic multisectoral roundtables were a factor in facilitating access. These were held between a variety of actors, including the Baja California State Board of Migratory Affairs, Baja California State Human Rights Commission (CEDHBC), IOM, United Nations High Commission for Refugees (UNHCR), Doctors Without Borders (in French, MSF), and local media outlets, though these apparently lacked the health jurisdiction.

Despite this, informants generally agreed that in practice, migrant access was restricted by significant barriers. No direct mechanisms were known that translated legislation into reality. A significant incongruence with the national legislation persisted within the obligatory online registry for vaccination, where as previously mentioned, in order to complete registration, individuals were required to provide a CURP number. In addition to the widespread challenge of online registration for migrants—most lack access to computers, though cell phones are common—the majority do not have a CURP number.

As described by a lawyer working with a CSO in the United States,

> [M]ost migrants do not have computers, so if the website doesn't work from a phone, they also wouldn't be able to access it. Additionally, in many places offering vaccines in Mexico, they are only offered to a specific population group at a time. There isn't always a lot of notice as to when a vaccine for your eligibility category will become available. I have not seen any government efforts to address information directly to migrants about vaccination. I have also not seen any governmental efforts to address misinformation about vaccines.

This testimony sheds light on the significant information and accessibility gaps faced by migrants, emphasising the urgent need for more inclusive and migrant-friendly vaccination campaign strategies.

Real access to healthcare services depended on the compliance of healthcare workers and adjacent personnel with the law; however, informants described discretionary actions by these gatekeepers as the main barrier to care. This was most commonly manifested in the widespread practice of healthcare workers asking for an official Mexican document, such as the CURP to provide services, although this is against the law. Some were reported to have even requested proof of migratory status and to have denied services to Afro-descendent, indigenous, or visibly non-Mexican individuals even if these persons showed valid documents.

In contrast to targeted mechanisms to reach the highly vulnerable migrant population, vaccination sites remained the main point of access, most of which were far from shelters, camps, and areas of high migrant concentration. This posed distance and cost barriers to vaccine access. Finally, the design of the overall COVID-19 vaccine campaign in Mexico created further challenges for migrants, as it did in other population groups. These campaigns have been characterised by their narrow specificity and unpredictability, where one particular group (e.g., adults 40–49 years old) were the only population at a given site on a given day, and notice was often very short and disseminated through non-standardised platforms.

Across the border in the United States, the federal government legally ensured open access to COVID-19 vaccines for all eligible individuals, regardless of their migratory status. This policy was reflected in the actions of state health actors and local governing bodies in the San Diego region, who vaccinated anyone presenting any form of valid identification. This approach was categorised as implementing low-level measures in accordance with the IOM 2021 standards.

The COVID-19 pandemic brought challenges well beyond the disease itself to public sector healthcare, with the complete closure of health centres for extended periods during 2020 and 2021. When open, limits were put on patient capacity, and certain installations, including Tijuana General Hospital, were converted to "COVID-19 only" spaces. The "covidisation" of healthcare limited the guarantee of other rights, such as sexual and reproductive rights (Vearey, Gruchy and Maple, 2021). Additionally, COVID-19 is far from the only relevant transmissible disease of the 21st century, as evidenced through examples like chickenpox outbreaks reported in shelters and in the *El Chaparral* camp (Hernández, 2021). Given the focus on COVID-19 and diversion from other health conditions, it is also important to continue to take action against non-communicable diseases, since the particular determinants of health lived by most migrants make them more vulnerable to these (Rubio, 2021).

In this challenging context, as the Chief of Operations at a Mexican CSO pointed out,

> [H]ealthcare services are provided by the health centre (which gave zero response in pandemic times), while the Tijuana General Hospital attends emergencies (this also stopped functioning completely during the pandemic since it was only for COVID-19 patients and had no available beds). We [in our organisation] have a medical clinic with volunteer personnel who care for any type of case presented. When a case is very serious, we call the Mexican Red Cross and pressure them until they either take care of the person or transfer them.

This underscores the dire circumstances faced by health services during the pandemic and the pivotal role played by civil society organisations in bridging healthcare gaps for marginalised groups like migrants.

Intergovernmental organisations, such as the IOM and the UNHCR, were reported to have significantly increased their presence in and around Tijuana since 2016. Though rarely providers of direct services, these organisations were central to general humanitarian assistance, resource distribution, legal and administrative accompaniment, COVID-19-related materials and services, and more. These organisations even provided critical pandemic resources to public sector hospitals with the aim of directly supporting not only migrants and refugees but also their host communities. As may be expected, international organisations were the actors perhaps most affected by pandemic-related US border closures, given the resulting limitations on transportation of people and materials.

The strong participation of international organisations like the IOM and the UNHCR highlights a collaborative, multi-actor approach fundamental to multistakeholder diplomacy. Their efforts are geared towards establishing integrated service delivery systems that are tailored to meet the needs of migrants, a primary goal of multistakeholder diplomacy for global health and migration. Furthermore, the active role of the IOM and UNHCR in the health and migration sectors serves not only as a prime example of multistakeholder diplomacy but also MLG.

The establishment of integrated service delivery systems, designed to meet the specific needs of migrants, exemplifies a combined multilevel and multistakeholder approach geared towards promoting both health and well-being (SDG 3) and reducing inequalities (SDG 10).

On the US side of the border, one informant highlighted community clinics and larger public sector agencies as service providers. The latter included state-level bodies like the California Department of Public Health and county-level bodies such as the San Diego County Health and Human Services Agency. This highlights a direct involvement of the government and therefore formal disease diplomacy, in contrast to reports from the Mexican side.

The direct participation of state-level organisations implies a hierarchical structure and centralised control, hallmarks of a centralist top-down governance style. The involvement of county-level agencies, exemplified by the San Diego County Health and Human Services Agency, points to a localist approach in governance, suggesting that policies and services are specifically tailored and executed at the territorial level.

Throughout the border region, though certain partnerships existed, informants noted a significant lack of formal alliances. Even when present, these were reportedly not designed to yield lasting impact. As a medical doctor and co-director of a CSO in Mexico observed, "*[T]he networks that have been established play a minimal role, functioning effectively only on the few occasions when government and NGO service brigades have collaborated, which, during the entire pandemic, amounted to merely two days.*" This comment underscores the sporadic and insufficient nature of these collaborative efforts in addressing the ongoing challenges of the pandemic.

The situation described earlier points towards a decoupled model of MLG, characterised by the absence of significant and sustained interactions, especially between governmental entities and NGOs. This lack of engagement reveals deficiencies in both formal and multi-stakeholder disease diplomacy, where established networks become effective only during infrequent instances of government-NGO collaboration. Ideally, these forms of diplomacy should foster sustainable and effective partnerships for addressing health crises like the COVID-19 pandemic.

According to Stoeva (2020), the WHO has emphasised that, particularly in the context of a pandemic, responses are more effective when rooted in cooperation and solidarity rather than isolated efforts and a mentality of self-preservation. This approach necessitates collaborative efforts from various stakeholders, including individuals, businesses (including healthcare providers), and community organisations. Such collaborations epitomise an ideal coordinated multistakeholder security policy, essential for effective management of global health emergencies.

Formal partnerships generally did not span the multiple sectors needed to ensure integral access and care but instead often consisted of strong ties among CSOs whose effectiveness and sustainability were often dependent on intersectoral partnerships. However, the limited capacity of CSOs to provide direct healthcare services made linkages with the Mexican public health sector a must. Informal and often unilateral relationships between CSOs and the public sector were widely recognised, but no formal partnerships were reported between the public sector and other actors.

As the director of a CSO in Mexico stated,

> [I]t is critical that governmental and social actors form partnerships to establish paths to access basic rights, such as health, and that individuals that need healthcare can receive dignified care independently of nationality, age, gender, migratory status, skin colour, ethnicity or any other characteristic that could provoke exclusionary practices. The reality in Tijuana is that few civil society spaces provide medical attention (free of charge) to communities in mobility, and there is no institutional response to the necessity and obligation of the state to provide care to those who need it. This situation directly harms the resources and capacities of individuals to adequately protect their own health.

This underscores the critical need for more established collaboration between civil society and government to address healthcare challenges effectively and bridge discretionary gaps in legislative compliance.

The close cross-border geographical and cultural ties across this international zone were a key part of informal and formal partnerships to facilitate resource distribution. These included ties between Mexican actors and CSOs and academic institutions in the United States. One US-based informant mentioned hearing repeatedly from his Mexican colleagues that without partnerships with individuals and organisations in California, practically no resources would be available for migrants in Tijuana.

However, in California, the partnerships were deemed equally necessary for the effective functioning of migrant health access in general and for COVID-19 vaccine distribution on the US side. For example, key partnerships between the Mexican Consulate in San Diego, San Diego public health services, and community organisations serving migrants helped organise vaccination sites that were geographically accessible to this population and which were capable of garnering the trust of this community.

As compared to other regions, factors that favoured partnerships in the Tijuana-San Diego region were also evident to participants. Tijuana has long been a reference point in Mexico and the wider Americas for the movement of people and goods. During the pandemic, its relevance to transnational trade worked in its favour in terms of broader COVID-19 vaccine access.

A professor and researcher in Mexico elaborated on this point, noting,

> In the city of Tijuana, our location at the border has greatly favoured our situation because the border was closed for the pandemic and that created an enormous pressure [to reopen it] due to the economic losses that this closure represented. So, from very early on—June 2021—there was a certain will for universal vaccination for those over 18 years

of age, including migrant individuals. Advances in vaccination [of the population] were a key factor in the negotiations to reopen the border.

This highlights how Tijuana's unique regional role influenced both the city's response to the pandemic and its vaccine distribution strategy, particularly regarding the inclusion of migrant populations.

Since the first reception of highly publicised "migrant caravans" in the years prior to the pandemic, the city has been a space of greater collaboration between actors. Though these caravans were not the first large groups of migrants transiting Mexico, their size, organisation, and media draw were unique in scale and fed unique socio-political responses.

A medical doctor and service coordinator at a CSO in Mexico highlighted this change, stating,

> More local and binational actors have organised and formed partnerships along the border to improve access to care for migrants since 2018, with the arrival of the first caravan. We saw more US and international volunteers and organisations providing aid to existing local organisations like Prevencasa, which expanded our resources and capabilities.

This testimony underscores the significant impact of the migrant caravans in fostering cooperation and strengthening networks across borders, particularly in enhancing healthcare services for migrants. For example, this phenomenon sparked the permanent installation of UN agencies such as the IOM and UNHCR in Tijuana.

Despite immense challenges, certain factors favoured healthcare access for migrants in Mexico during the COVID-19 pandemic. Interestingly, sensitisation around COVID-19 at a global level benefitted migrant access to vaccines, though this did not extend to general healthcare service access. Given the weak presence of the state, informants described new linkages that served to obtain resources through innovative fundraising schemes and electronic transfers (Del Monte and McKee Irwin, 2020). The support came not only from international organisations but also from foundations, academic institutions, and populations (Ramírez-Meda and Moreno-Guitiérrez, 2020). Informants agreed that the global attention to COVID-19 provoked a temporary surge in donations, mainly from organisations and individuals in the United States to CSOs in Mexico. Some Mexican migrant shelters benefitted from the reception of vaccines through partnerships with organisations in San Diego and other places in the United States, though vaccine supply for migrants was still seen as dependent on convenience.

Another positive aspect of the pandemic in terms of partnerships was, for some informants, an increase in dialogue between Mexican state actors and CSOs serving migrants. This was seen to have improved over the course of the pandemic and in spite of serious initial challenges, though it was still insufficient for the depth of need. One participant also noted that the widespread normalisation of virtual meetings greatly facilitated collaboration with actors both near and far.

Unfortunately, and as may be expected, the pandemic also brought significant obstacles to partnerships, particularly cross-border collaboration. Facets of the pandemic itself directly hindered services and interactions, such as the conversion of healthcare centres to provide care only to COVID-19 patients and the contagion of healthcare workers themselves and their subsequent inability to provide services. Lack of political will from the Mexican public health sector to collaborate with other actors was described by several participants who, even as key civil society actors, were not included in any public sector actions for migrant care.

A medical doctor and co-director of a CSO in Mexico remarked,

> I have not personally witnessed any government efforts to provide vaccines to migrants. This does not mean that they didn't exist, but if they did, they were not widely publicised and they did not seek to involve many civil society groups in direct contact with migrants.

This comment highlights a disconnect between public health initiatives and the on-the-ground needs and efforts of civil society organisations dedicated to migrant care.

The hearts of most CSOs on both sides of the border are volunteers, both medical and non-medical. Fewer volunteers due to COVID-19 prevention measures had a devastating impact on CSO services by limited organisational capacity, sometimes causing the complete suspension of operations. A professor in the United States elaborated on this situation, stating,

> At the beginning of the pandemic, when orders were given to stay at home on both sides of the border, the many volunteers that used to serve migrant communities, including those from the medical sector, had to stop their normal activities. With time, services have begun to be re-established, since several months ago I would say they're back to normal, but particularly before the vaccines (that is, before vaccines were made available to volunteers), the volunteers stopped reporting.

This account highlights the critical role volunteers play in sustaining CSO operations and the significant challenges they faced during the pandemic, particularly before the widespread availability of COVID-19 vaccines.

These volunteer mobilisations and adaptive responses of CSOs to the COVID-19 crisis exemplify key elements of informal disease diplomacy. These actions, beyond the realm of formal governmental structures, are heavily dependent on the initiative and engagement of civil society and community groups. However, this approach has its limitations. The decrease in volunteer involvement and scarcity of resources during the pandemic underscores the inherent challenges of relying exclusively on informal diplomacy during global health crises. This situation underscores the need for a more integrated and robust framework that can effectively combine local initiatives with broader support systems to comprehensively address crises.

The halt in cross-border collaboration significantly affected various sectors, notably impeding research activities that could have provided valuable insights into the experiences of migration and health during the pandemic. This impact was acutely felt in the academic sphere, as shared by an informant from a university in the United States:

> [M]y university forbade us from travelling for research activities for more than 15 months. Although we performed some mini projects using remote instruments during the pandemic, we are just barely starting a deep-dive investigation about the experiences of migrants in Tijuana during the pandemic.

This comment from the professor highlights the challenges faced by researchers in gathering first-hand data during the pandemic, especially in cross-border contexts, which could otherwise inform decision-makers at multiple levels. The inability to travel further confines studies to remote methodologies, restricting the scope and depth necessary for thorough research with hard-to-reach populations like migrants. This reveals a critical need for both formal and multistakeholder diplomacy capable of navigating the challenges presented by global emergencies, such as the pandemic. A more formalised framework of cooperation, encompassing governments, academic institutions, and international organisations, could have significantly aided in sustaining vital research activities despite prevailing travel constraints.

Around San Diego, the response to the pandemic was considered overall to be efficient and collaborative, including public sector actors at the state and local level, as well as community organisations. In the view of one participant, this collaboration enabled a quick and effective pandemic response for the public, which generally extended to migrants. Considering this, it is clear that in the field of migration and with respect to the 2030 Agenda, a multiplicity of actors and sectors must intervene: governmental and non-governmental, international and local, and more. Local groups may include not only grassroots organisations but also volunteer groups.

The challenges faced in fully realising SDGs 3 and 10 during the COVID-19 pandemic underscore the urgent need for an integrated approach that spans multiple levels of governance and encompasses a comprehensive multi-stakeholder diplomatic strategy. Such approaches must be tailored not only to mitigate the immediate health impacts of the pandemic but also to address the deep-rooted systemic inequalities that have been prominently highlighted by this crisis.

However, it is evident that efforts in 2020–2021, while contributing to some extent towards achieving SDGs 3 and 10, fell short. This shortfall was largely due to the nature of the pandemic that has laid bare the inadequacies in the current system, revealing a critical need for more concerted and effective measures beyond addressing health issues in isolation and instead tackling the broader spectrum of contributing social and economic disparities.

The situation at the Tijuana-San Diego border region illustrates the complex layers of vulnerability, especially in healthcare access among migrants. Informants considered that any migrant, independent of other characteristics, was vulnerable to inadequate healthcare access. Nevertheless, a variety of intrinsic and extrinsic characteristics were clearly linked to greater relative vulnerability. Gender proved to be an important determinant, where women were almost unanimously considered to be the group of greatest concern, particularly when they also experienced other layers of vulnerability.

This is starkly illustrated by a professor and researcher from Mexico who observed,

> In Tijuana, without a doubt, the fragility of many women alone and with children is very notable. It makes no difference where they come from, whether from Central America or even from other parts of Mexico; for the purposes of vulnerability and the threat of multiple acts of violence it doesn't matter. . . There's no doubt that these sectors are extremely vulnerable [and particularly] where COVID-19 was a big factor.

This highlights how the pandemic has intensified existing challenges and exposed migrant women to additional risks.

Pregnant women in particular were also deemed a neglected group, especially in terms of prenatal care. According to Méndez (2020), "[T]here are no specialised protocols for the medical and psychological care of pregnant women and those with special needs" (Méndez, 2020, p. 51). This was emphasised by a lawyer from a US-based CSO, who shared a distressing example:

> Among migrants who are pregnant, I have seen a consistent lack of access to prenatal care apart from what non-profit organisations are able to provide. One of our clients lost a pregnancy at 7 months because the baby needed immediate neonatal surgical treatment and was unable to receive it. However, had this woman had access to prenatal care, this problem likely could have been caught months earlier.

This underscores the critical gaps in healthcare provision for pregnant migrant women, where an absence of targeted care can lead to severe, preventable consequences.

In contrast, one informant highlighted men as a notably vulnerable gender since they overwhelmingly form the group of migrants who are "returned" from the United States and live on the streets of Tijuana. As the professor and researcher from Mexico noted,

> I'd say that the situation of "migrants" in general is difficult . . . It's impossible to say that the situation of deported people is much better

[than that of women]. On the contrary, many of them were kicked out of the U.S. from one day to the next after living there 20 years, and after a few months in Tijuana it's not unusual to see them living in the street.

This statement sheds light on the harsh realities faced by many male migrants, particularly those who have been deported to Mexico.

Deportation from the United States was strongly linked to indigency in Tijuana and, therefore, to difficulties in healthcare access. Returnees included both Mexicans and non-Mexicans, particularly during the pandemic in the form of indiscriminate expedited returns under Title 42.[2] US asylum seekers confined to Mexico under the so-called US Migration Protection Protocols (MPP), also known as "Remain in Mexico" (*Quédate en México*),[3] also lacked health access in Mexico. This group, overwhelmingly male, generally lacked the basic conditions necessary to ensure safety and health, including housing and social support. This highlights a grave aspect of gender-based vulnerability experienced by males.

The lesbian, gay, bisexual, transgender, queer, and other members of the LGBTQ+ community were also noted as subject to harsh discrimination, which affected healthcare access and other critical areas. The lack of migratory documents in Mexico was another strong determinant of vulnerability and led to a series of further negative consequences, including the lack of inscription in the Mexican public sector health system (since 2018, INSABI, and since 2023, IMSS Bienestar).

Age was also reported to affect vulnerability, as children and adolescents were of special concern to informants, particularly when unaccompanied. According to Méndez, "civil society organisations in border areas have documented expulsions of this group to Mexico, in addition to other irregularities in the actions of the authorities" (Méndez, 2020, p. 51). For example, the lack of a protocol to monitor returnees or the non-negotiation between the Instituto Nacional de Migración (INM) (National Institute for Migration) and US authorities that would orchestrate deportations at times that guarantee health screenings and humanitarian attention (El COLEF, 2020). This lack of a protocol affects binational health security. This weakness in the health field is tied to the institutional and systemic level because unilateral measures were taken during the administration of US President Donald Trump, which affected the functioning of the US-Mexico Border Health Commission (BHC) (Moya, Coronado and Mumme, 2021).

In a healthcare context often characterised as xenophobic and racist, migrant race and culture played an important role in healthcare access. Central Americans—including Salvadorans, Guatemalans, Hondurans, and Nicaraguans—were subject to greater limitations, as were afro-descendants, including Haitians.

The director of one Mexican CSO explained:

Migrants who are foreigners [not Mexicans] are those who experience the most vulnerability when it comes to healthcare access, since they do not have migratory documents and they are denied Mexican public healthcare services. It's also important to mention that when these individuals try to access their right to health, those of Haitian or African origin fall victim to racism by the same institutions, which in many cases do not even check whether people have migratory documents or not. They deny them access anyway.

This reveals a systemic issue in healthcare access, particularly highlighting how the lack of migratory documentation disproportionately affects non-Mexican migrants, leading to their exclusion from public healthcare services. This situation is further exacerbated for migrants of Haitian or African origin, who face additional barriers due to institutional racism. Such discrimination is prevalent even without verification of their migratory status, indicating a deeply ingrained bias in the healthcare system. This underscores the urgent need for policy reforms and public awareness initiatives to combat discriminatory practices and ensure equitable healthcare access for all migrants, regardless of their origin or documentation status.

One researcher from Mexico further emphasised this, stating, "*[In]n Tijuana we've seen through our fieldwork that in some clinics rejection of the migrant population is widespread and attributable to a xenophobic environment, especially with individuals who are Central American or extra-continental and do not speak Spanish.*" These insights bring to light the multifaceted challenges that migrants face, particularly those rooted in racial and cultural biases, further emphasising the critical need for inclusive and non-discriminatory healthcare practices. The vulnerability of non-Spanish-speaking migrants is particularly acute, as they often lack access to verifiable information and are more susceptible to misinformation and disinformation.

Mexican migrants in Tijuana (often from the states of Guerrero, Michoacán, or Chiapas) still confront significant barriers to healthcare access. This highlights the social condition of migrants as a factor that alone can transcend nationality and even migratory status. Institutional discrimination and unequal access to medical care reflect shortcomings in formal disease diplomacy, where government policies and actions should guarantee the right to health for all, regardless of their migratory status or ethnicity.

This also demonstrates a decoupled governance model, characterised by a disconnect between healthcare policies formulated at the national level and their implementation at the local level, a problem that is particularly acute in areas with high migrant populations. This disconnect leads to inconsistent and incoherent healthcare services, further intensifying the difficulties migrants face in accessing necessary medical care. These disparities underscore the urgent need for a more integrated and coordinated approach to governance to effectively close the gap between policy development and practical application in healthcare delivery.

This need for alignment is further highlighted by frequent discriminatory acts against migrants reported around Tijuana. As the director of a Mexican CSO pointed out,

> Communities in the mobility context have been those most impacted during the pandemic, because beyond just lacking economic resources, they overwhelmingly face discriminatory and racist practices which serve to deny them healthcare services, both in general and in services related to COVID-19.

This emphasises systemic issues in the application of healthcare policies and the need for reforms to ensure equitable and non-discriminatory healthcare access.

Some mechanisms for healthcare access are present at international, binational, national, and local levels in Mexico. At the international level, different mechanisms were designed to guide actors, especially governments, in adopting measures to "leave no one behind" (the motto of the 2030 Agenda) during the pandemic. This pertains especially to groups at risk. The guidance document *COVID-19 and the Human Rights of Migrants: Guidance of the OHCHR* indicates that "migrants can be particularly vulnerable to stigma and discrimination and can be excluded in law, policy and practice from access to rights, including in the context of the public health and recovery response to COVID-19" (OHCHR, 2020, p. 1).

In the United States, national guidelines by governmental actors to improve vaccination, guarantee health security, and guide action to address the migratory phenomenon. The National Strategic Vaccine Plan (2021–2025) was designed to provide a "roadmap for federal and non-federal partners and stakeholders for strengthening vaccination infrastructure across public and private sectors, including the improvement of immunisation and health equity. Its aim is to prevent vaccine-preventable diseases" (HHS, 2021, p. 4) and "ensure its own national health security" (HHS, 2021, p. 12). Although there is no explicit reference to groups at risk in this plan, one of its strategies is oriented towards sociodemographic factors (racial and ethnic, age, disability, social, economic, cultural, and other types) that contribute to vaccination disparities (Strategy 4.2.1). Data from HHS 2021 show that in the United States there were low immunisation rates among children living in poverty, children enrolled in Medicaid, and black children; among adults, immunisation coverage was generally lower among non-Hispanic blacks, Hispanics, and non-Hispanic Asians compared to non-Hispanic whites (HHS, 2021).

For Ross *et al.* (2021), these differences are linked to federal immigration policies. For example, not having a legal documentation status is a determinant that influences the experience of migrants in healthcare access. On the other hand, modification of policies is not sufficient to eliminate the prevailing fear of deportation in the undocumented migrant community, and significant communication actions must be carried out in different languages to combat mistrust towards the public sphere (Ross *et al.*, 2021).

In Mexico, several guidelines were created, including the National Vaccination Policy against the SARS-CoV-2 Virus for the Prevention of COVID-19 and the Operational Plan for the Care of the Migrant Population during COVID-19. Version 6.0 (May 2021) of the National Policy explicitly references migrants as priority groups in vaccination campaigns. Furthermore, it states that nationality, migration status, and the lack of official identity documents (birth certificate, voter ID, CURP, passport, or others) should not limit access (Gobierno de México, 2021). However, this national policy has not been translated into a real guarantee of healthcare services.

Regarding the Operational Plan, lines of action are established to provide comprehensive healthcare to migrants (pre-hospital, primary, and secondary care levels). This is hierarchical and based on a model of top-down relationships, from the government down to non-governmental organisations, since the central coordination of the provision of healthcare is the responsibility of the state, local health services (SESA), and the health jurisdictions of the border zones and along the migratory route. According to this document, coordination would not exclude a link with different instances of the health sector, the INM, NGOs, and state and municipal governments. There has also been a need to build more effective relationships with migrant shelters. To achieve this, one objective of the Operational Plan is to inventory the services provided and the risk factors (overcrowding, resources, and response capacity) that increase the spread of the disease within facilities (Gobierno de México. Secretaría de Salud, n.d.).

Beyond what is proposed in this plan, operational gaps are evident, since a lack of financial resources has diluted the role of local governments in caring for this population during the pandemic. This was in part an effect of the austerity policy of current Mexican President Andrés López Obrador. One measure adopted was the elimination of the Migrant Support Fund (in Spanish, FAM) from the Mexican federal budget, whose resources were put towards the operating expenses of some CSOs (Guerrero, 2019; Ramírez-Meda and Moreno-Guitiérrez, 2020). Other factors that influenced shelter operations were border closures by the United States for non-essential travel and social distancing measures adopted in both countries. Border closures placed significant strains on the provision of in-kind services and support, which rely heavily on charitable donations, mostly from the United States (Del Monte and McKee Irwin, 2020).

At the binational level, there are risk reduction mechanisms for the protection of the population. According to Menzel (2020), Mexico and the United States "have implemented a series of measures to jointly address health risks of mutual interest" (Menzel, 2020, p. 131). One of these measures is the BHC, which aims to "identify and evaluate public health problems that precede the border population" (Menzel, 2020, p. 131) "by engaging local, state, federal, and international leaders to collaborate with health professionals" (Velasco, 2014, p. 83). Among its most notable initiatives are the US-Mexico Border Tuberculosis Consortium and the Border Binational Health Week (Velasco, 2014). The week later expanded to the whole month of October and included "numerous health promotion and disease prevention activities on both sides of the border." On the other hand, "Leaders Across Borders (LAB) is an advanced leadership development program aimed at building the binational leadership capacity of public health, health care, and other community professionals working to improve the health of communities in the U.S.-Mexico border region" (HHS, 2021).

In San Diego and Tijuana, initiatives also exist in the framework of health security for the border control of tuberculosis (TB). An example of this is "the International Community Foundation, which is the fiscal sponsor of the Bridges of Hope Program. . . . Its main functions are to facilitate laboratory testing of individuals from Baja California in San Diego, California; administering anti-TB medications for patients from that state of Mexico; supplying specialised personnel to monitor anti-TB therapy there; and creating a binational network of experts" (Valle, 2014, p. 101).

There are also initiatives that transcend the governmental sphere, such as the Binational Health Collaboration Program implemented by the US-Mexico Foundation for Science (FUMEC) and the US-Mexico Border Philanthropy Partnership (BPP). While the first aims to "improve Mexican epidemiological tracking systems with resources from the U.S. State and Health and Human Services Departments, as well as the Centers for Disease Control and Prevention (CDC)" (Valle, 2014, p. 100), the second includes leaders and organisations from academia, business and corporate entities, government, philanthropy, and non-profit organisations. The BPP supported the launch of the first binational committee to promote philanthropy and citizen participation and, in September 2018, signed a memorandum of understanding with the Mexico section of the BHC and the Consulate General of Mexico in San Diego to provide technical assistance for the provision of healthcare services through the *Ventanillas de Salud* (Health Windows) and Wellness programmes.

However, the lack of effective mechanisms to ensure healthcare access for migrants was a common theme among informants. As a professor in the United Nations pointed out,

"Guarantee" doesn't seem like the correct word. There are different mechanisms, each of which declare their intent to facilitate healthcare access for migrants of different profiles. But that doesn't guarantee anything, particularly for those migrants who are more vulnerable including not only those who are living in the street, but also those who do not speak Spanish (migrants who speak Haitian Creole, indigenous languages, English or French).

This sheds light on the inadequacy of current systems and the need for more robust, effective strategies to ensure equitable healthcare access for all migrants, particularly those facing compounded vulnerabilities due to language barriers and living conditions.

This issue was compounded by a pervasive "Mexicans first" attitude, extending within and beyond COVID-19-related care. A medical doctor and service coordinator from a CSO in Mexico attributed this to the overall inadequacy of the health system:

> Our public system is far beyond capacity, staff is insufficient, overworked and underpaid and there are simply not enough resources to sometimes provide just basic care. So, there are no clear or functioning mechanisms to address xenophobia, racism and discrimination from public servants besides filing a complaint, which many avoid and when done yields little results or fails to leave any lasting impact.

This highlights systemic issues within the public health system that exacerbate discriminatory practices, indicating a need for systemic reform to ensure equitable healthcare access. The prioritisation of Mexicans and discrimination in access to healthcare services demonstrate failures by the actors involved in formal disease diplomacy.

Some informants agreed that many barriers confronted by migrants in the health system were encountered by Mexicans as well, noting particularly that sometimes discrimination could be explained not only by anti-migrant discrimination but also against the poor. However, it was made clear that actions directed specifically towards migrants placed a significant barrier before healthcare and COVID-19 vaccine access, and that the Mexican public sector was a perpetrator rather than a defender.

This perspective is further elucidated by a Mexican professor and researcher who noted:

> There are many, many [cases of discrimination]. I wrote an article recently where I explained the contradictions within a country such as Mexico, where we asked those who formed part of the migrant caravans for all their medical tests and certificates to confirm that they weren't bringing a virus, but at the same time the travellers that arrived by aeroplane weren't asked for anything, demonstrating a fundamentally racist and classist rationale.

This underscores the systemic nature of discrimination within the health system.

As with COVID-19 vaccination misinformation, this systemic discrimination seemed to heavily impact the perception by migrants of their rights in

Mexico, despite what the law says. A lawyer from a US-based CSO elaborated on this, stating:

> [G]enerally speaking, xenophobia and racism against migrants always play a role in access to healthcare. Even if people haven't necessarily had a bad experience with the Mexican authorities or healthcare institutions themselves, they definitely know someone else who has. So even in situations where someone is theoretically eligible to receive treatment, they might not even try because of past experiences or what they have heard from others.

This highlights how the collective experiences and perceptions of discrimination can deter migrant individuals from seeking healthcare services, even when they are legally entitled to them. More inclusive and migrant-friendly healthcare policies and practices, as well as effective communication strategies to ensure migrants are knowledgeable and empowered to exercise their rights, are solutions.

Not only direct discriminatory practices but also the lack of protective mechanisms against them was recognised to cause significant damage. No campaigns were known to exist that targeted migrants to provide reliable information about healthcare service access or the COVID-19 vaccine, much less to fight misinformation known to be rampant within widely used social network channels. No translation services were readily available for non-Spanish speakers—a migrant group noted to suffer the most significant barriers to service access—nor were healthcare personnel trained in intersectionality, interculturality, or trauma management.

In the San Diego area, informants reported no direct discriminatory practices. Nonetheless, Ambrosio (2021) and others have noted similarities to Mexico in the reasons behind the lack of effective access for certain migrant groups, including lack of English language skills, limited financial access to health services, absence of a Social Security Number (SSN), and inadequate communication campaigns. Although migrants in San Diego are eligible to receive free COVID-19 vaccination, local organisations have highlighted that the measures implemented have not been enough to gain the trust of this population; for example, when scheduling an appointment on the portal, an SSN was requested. This measure discouraged registration, despite the fact that the portal indicated that if you did not have an SSN, you could enter "000–00–0000" (Mendoza, 2021).

For migrants in the United States, faulty information was also at the heart of access issues during the pandemic. In particular, systematising information was a challenge that affected the awareness and availability of migrant individuals to register for the vaccine. Furthermore, this was noted as affecting the ability of migrants to access testing, forming a notable difference as compared to Mexico, where testing was not mentioned as a primary issue.

This is likely due to the lack of widespread and affordable testing options for the general Mexican public as compared to the US context.

The prevalent issue of unequal access to medical care and entrenched discriminatory practices within the health systems of the region stands in stark opposition to SDG 3. Achieving this necessitates systemic reforms and the adoption of inclusive policies. The failure of the health system and government to enforce policies that provide equitable health rights to all, regardless of their nationality or ethnic background, clearly contradicts the objectives of SDG 10. This goal aims not just to foster equal opportunities but also to diminish inequalities in outcomes by eradicating discriminatory laws, policies, and practices. Consequently, advancing towards the fulfilment of SDG 10 demands urgent attention to these shortcomings in healthcare access and a concerted effort to dismantle systemic bias and discrimination. Such a strategic approach would enhance equity in healthcare access and significantly contribute to reducing national and global inequalities, ensuring just and inclusive treatment for everyone.

The gap between policy intentions and actual healthcare delivery, especially in terms of equitable access, belies a decoupled governance model. This disconnect is seen in the failure to implement inclusive health policies effectively at different levels of governance, from local to national. The discrimination against certain groups around healthcare access demonstrates failures in formal disease diplomacy. This is where government-led initiatives and international cooperation should work towards inclusive health policies that align with global health goals such as SDGs 3, 10, and 17.

Conclusion

The objective of this chapter was to analyse the dynamics of cooperation among various actors in the US-Mexico border region of San Diego-Tijuana in relation to facilitating access to COVID-19-related healthcare and vaccination for migrants during the pandemic in 2020–2021.

Disease diplomacy emerged as a key analytical framework, highlighting the importance of international cooperation and MLG in public-sector health management in border regions. The findings indicate that interactions between state, intergovernmental, and non-state actors were fundamental but weak, where significant challenges were revealed in implementing policies and maintaining sustainable and effective partnerships.

CSOs and NGOs played a crucial role in bridging the gap between migrant communities and the public healthcare sector. The involvement of international organisations such as IOM and UNHCR underscores the importance of a multistakeholder approach in disease diplomacy. However, responses were marked by a lack of coordination and significant institutional and logistical barriers.

Institutional discrimination and unequal practices in accessing healthcare services were constant, reflecting failures in formal disease diplomacy. These barriers were manifested in the inability to apply health policies equitably, exacerbating existing inequalities. The need for systemic reforms and inclusive policies was evident to meet the SDGs, especially SDG 3 (well-being) and 10 (reduction of inequalities).

This chapter explored a disconnect between national-level health policies and their implementation at the local level, particularly in a region with high migrant mobility. This decoupled governance model underscores the need for a more integrated and coordinated governance approach. Multistakeholder diplomacy and partnerships between different sectors and levels of governance were fundamental, though often insufficient to meet needs.

COVID-19 can be considered a pandemic of inequalities, in which migrants have been one of the most disadvantaged groups not only due to health measures but also due to policies such as MPP and Title 42, which directly impact orderly migration. The border has become an endless waiting room.

Systemic factors that differentiate the experiences of migrants in accessing COVID-19 vaccines, some of which are in Mexico and the United States, may be categorised as low- to medium-level administrative barriers. Informants identified that one barrier in Mexico is the need for a personal identification number, also known as CURP, while in the United States it is the SSN. Requiring this type of documentation does not reduce inequalities, nor does it contribute to the motto of the 2030 Agenda of leaving no one behind.

To achieve the SDGs, especially in the context of global health crises like the COVID-19 pandemic, a more robust and coordinated approach is needed that combines local initiatives with broader support systems. Systemic reforms, formalised cooperation among diverse actors, and the implementation of inclusive and non-discriminatory health policies are essential to ensure equitable access to healthcare and reduce health inequalities. To achieve the 2030 Agenda, it is critical to break with the silos that "covidisation" has generated and guided essential goods and services towards border risk factors for migrants from a differentiated, intersectional, intercultural, lifecycle, gender, and human rights approach.

In summary, this chapter underscores the complexity of health responses in border contexts during the pandemic and highlights the urgent need for a more effective MLG and integrative disease diplomacy to address health inequalities and advance towards the achievement of SDGs 3, 10, and 17.

Notes

1 The authors are grateful to their research assistants at the Universidad Iberoamericana Mexico City for their work in reviewing literature and identifying key elements based on analysis variables: Ximena Bailón, Daniela Martínez, and Jessica Quezada.
2 Title 42 is a public health and welfare statute enacted in 1944 that serves as an instrument to determine whether a communicable disease in a foreign country poses a serious danger of spreading into the United States, either by people or goods entering the country. During the pandemic, this instrument has been used to control migratory movements (Castillo and Garcia, 2021).

3 This measure, announced by the US government in 2018 and formally implemented in Mexico in 2019, forced asylum seekers to await the resolution of their cases in Mexican territory. According to the Institute for Women in Migration (in Spanish, IMUMI), "[O]n the American side, it has been implemented in San Diego and Calexico, California; and in El Paso, Brownsville, Laredo and Eagle Pass, Texas. On the Mexican side, the return is made in the neighbouring cities" (IMUMI, 2019, p. 3) such as Tijuana, Mexicali and Ciudad Juárez. For Ramírez-Meda and Moreno-Guitiérrez (2020), these cities can be considered "waiting rooms."

References

Agudo, A. (2020) 'Actores clave en Baja California. Instituciones públicas, albergues, organizaciones de la sociedad civil y movimientos sociales en torno a la migración', in *Desafíos y riesgos enfrentados por albergues, organizaciones civiles y personas migrantes en Tijuana 2019, Una propuesta de diálogo desde la Universidad Iberoamericana*. Tijuana: Ibero, pp. 39–72.

Ambrosio, R. (2021) *Acceso a los servicios de salud de connacionales en Estados Unidos y en el momento de su retorno a México*. Gaceta—Facultad de Medicina. [Online]. Available at: https://gaceta.facmed.unam.mx/index.php/2021/05/06/acceso-a-los-servicios-de-salud-de-connacionales-en-estados-unidos-y-en-el-momento-de-su-retorno-a-mexico/ (Accessed 12 January 2024).

Barragán, J.C., Riaño, M.I. and Martínez, M. (2012) 'Redes integradas de servicios de salud: hacia la construcción de un concepto', *Revista Universidad y Salud*, 14(2), pp. 186–196.

Castillo, A. and Garcia, K. (2021) 'El Título 42 explicado: La oscura política de salud pública en el centro de una lucha fronteriza de Estados Unidos', *Los Angeles Times*. [Online]. Available at: www.latimes.com/espanol/eeuu/articulo/2021-10-28/que-es-el-titulo-42-como-afecta-a-la-inmigracion-fronteriza-de-los-norteameri canos (Accessed 12 January 2024).

Castro-Conde, C. (2010) 'A vueltas con la "gobernanza multinivel', *Revista Española de Ciencia Política*, 22, pp. 119–133.

Davies, S.E., Kamradt-Scott, A. and Rushton, S. (2015) *Disease diplomacy: international norms and global health security*. Baltimore: John Hopkins University Press.

Del Monte, J.A. and McKee Irwin, R. (2020) *Personas Migrantes en Tijuana frente al COVID-19: Impactos y consecuencias de las medidas sanitarias desde la perspectiva de los actores*. Global Migration Center (UC Davis), Observatorio de Legislación y Política Migratoria (El COLEF).

Economic Commission for Latin America and the Caribbean (ECLAC) (2018) *Guía metodológica: planificación para la implementación de la Agenda 2030 en América Latina y el Caribe*. Santiago: ECLAC.

El Colegio de la Frontera Norte (EL COLEF) (2020) *Poblaciones vulnerables ante el COVID-19. Personas migrantes en Tijuana frente al COVID-19: Impactos y consecuencias de las medidas sanitarias desde la perspectiva de los actores*. [Online]. Available at: www.colef.mx/estudiosdeelcolef/personas-migrantes-en-tijuana-frente-al-covid-19-impactos-y-consecuencias-de-las-medidas-sanitarias-desde-la-perspectiva-de-los-actores/ (Accessed 12 January 2024).

Gobierno de México (2021) 'Política nacional rectora de vacunación contra el SARS-CoV-2 para la prevención de la COVID-19 en México. Documento rector. National Vaccination Policy against the SARS-COV-2 Virus, for the prevention of COVID-19 in Mexico', *Governing Document*. 11 May. [Online]. Available at: https://coronavirus.gob.mx/wp-content/uploads/2021/05/11May2021_PNVx_COVID.pdf (Accessed 12 January 2024).

Gobierno de México. Secretaría de Salud (n.d.) *Preparación y respuesta frente a casos de SARS-CoV2-2019 para la atención primaria de la salud*. [Online]. Available at: https://coronavirus.gob.mx/wp-content/uploads/2020/04/Preparacion_respuesta_casos_SARS-CoV2_atencion_primaria.pdf (Accessed 12 January 2024).

Guerrero, J. (2019) 'Gobierno de AMLO desapareció Fondo de Apoyo a Migrantes; deja en desamparo a migrantes oaxaqueños', *Redacción Oaxaca*. [Online]. Available at: https://redaccionoaxaca.com/index.php/2019/01/01/gobierno-de-amlo-desaparecio-fondo-de-apoyo-a-migrantes-deja-en-desamparo-a-migrantes-oaxaq uenos/ (Accessed 12 January 2024).

Hernández, J.M. (2021) 'Mantienen cerco de migrantes por brote de varicela', *El Sol de México, Citing El Sol de Tijuana*, 28 July. [Online]. Available at: www.elsol demexico.com.mx/republica/sociedad/mantienen-cerco-de-migrantes-por-brote-de-varicela-7015530.html (Accessed 12 January 2024).

Hooghe, L. and Marks, G. (2002) 'Types of multi-level governance', *Les Cahiers européens de Sciences Po*, 3, pp. 1–32.

Hooghe, L. and Marks, G. (2003) 'Unraveling the central state, but how? Types of multilevel governance', *American Political Science Review*, 97(2), pp. 233–243.

Institute for Women in Migration (IMUMI) (2019) *Recursos para entender el Protocolo 'Quédate en México*. [Online]. Available at: https://imumi.org/attachments/2019/Recursos-para-entender-el-Protocolo2019.pdf (Accessed 12 January 2024).

International Organization for Migration (IOM) (2015) *World migration report 2015*. Switzerland: IOM.

International Organization for Migration (IOM) (2021) *Migrant inclusion in COVID-19 vaccination campaigns*. [Online]. Available at: https://drive.google.com/file/d/1YtYNbxNxS681r1MSpeEuQXdhCehdNTJ5/view (Accessed 12 January 2024).

Katz, R. *et al.* (2011) 'Defining health diplomacy: changing demands in the era of globalization', *The Milbank Quarterly*, 89(3).

Libert-Amico, A. *et al.* (2018) 'Experiencias de gobernanza multinivel en México: innovación para la reducción de emisiones de carbono de los ecosistemas terrestres', *Madera y Bosques*, 24, pp. 1–18.

Méndez, M. (coord.) (2020) *Informe sobre los efectos de la pandemia de COVID-19 en las personas migrantes y refugiadas*. Mexico City: CMDPDH.

Mendoza, A. (2021) 'San Diego ofrece la vacuna contra COVID-19 a residentes indocumentados, estos lidian con la desconfianza', *The San Diego Union-Tribune*. [Online]. Available at: www.sandiegouniontribune.com/en-espanol/primera-plana/articulo/2021-02-01/vacuna-indocumentados (Accessed 12 January 2024).

Menzel, C. (2020) 'Pandemias, epidemias y seguridad', in Lozano, A. and Rodríguez, A. (coords.) *Seguridad y asuntos internacionales*. Mexico: Asociación Mexicana de Estudios Internacionales (AMEI), Siglo XXI Editores, pp. 125–135.

Moya, E., Coronado, I. and Mumme, S. (2021) 'A call to action: reestablishment of the U.S.-Mexico border health commission', *More Than A Magazine, A Movement*. [Online]. Available at: https://drive.google.com/file/d/13bEhSYpBaCzgDPJH ewNZZ2BRnSCXRPOW/view (Accessed 12 January 2024).

Müller, P. (2014) *La contribución de las Organizaciones de la Sociedad Civil a la defensa de los derechos humanos de migrantes en la región fronteriza Tijuana-Mexicali-San Diego, 1994–2014*. Mexico: El Colegio de la Frontera Norte.

Office of the High Commissioner for Human Rights (OHCHR) (2020) *COVID-19 and the human rights of migrants: guidance*. [Online]. Available at: www.ohchr.org/Documents/Issues/Migration/OHCHRGuidance_COVID19_Migrants.pdf (Accessed 12 January 2024).

Ortega, A. (2021) 'Ciudades y migrantes, tensiones entre gobernanza, derecho internacional y gestión. Odisea', *Revista de Estudios Migratorios*, 8, pp. 76–101.

Panizzon, M. and van Riemsdijk, M. (2019) 'Introduction to special issue: "migration governance in an era of large movements: a multi-level approach"', *Journal of Ethnic and Migration Studies*, 45(8), pp. 1225–1241.

Porras, F. (2021) 'La metagobernanza y las alianzas de múltiples interesados', in Sosa, G. and Ayala, C. (coords.) *Alianzas para el desarrollo y la instrumentación de la Agenda 2030*. Mexico City: Instituto de Investigaciones Dr. José María Luis Mora, pp. 23–46.

Quiroga, G. (2019) *Características de los servicios de salud y factores sociodemográficos que influyen en la utilización de los mismos, de la población del área urbana de conocoto en el período 2015-2016*. Disertación previa a la obtención del titulo de médico cirujano. Pontificia Universidad Católica del Ecuador.

Ramírez, A.L. (2021) 'Sin resultados, el Centro Integrador Migrante Carmen Serdán', *El Sol de Tijuana*, 12 July. [Online]. Available at: www.elsoldetijuana.com.mx/local/sin-resultados-el-centro-integrador-migrante-carmen-serdan-6952106.html (Accessed 12 January 2024).

Ramírez-Meda, K.M. and Moreno-Guitiérrez, A.T. (2020) 'Los albergues para migrantes en México, frente al COVID-19: el caso de Mexicali, Baja California', *Huellas de la migración*, 5(10), pp. 39–59.

Risse, T. (2011) 'Governance in areas of limited statehood: introduction and overview', in Risse, T. (ed.) *Governance without state? Policies and politics in areas of limited statehood*. New York: Columbia University Press, pp. 1–35.

Ross, H.M. *et al.* (2021) 'U.S. immigration policies pose threat to health security during COVID-19 pandemic', *Health Security*, 19(S1), pp. 83–88.

Rubio, V. (2021) *Análisis del panorama de la salud en la frontera norte de México*. Gaceta—Facultad de Medicina. [Online]. Available at: https://gaceta.facmed.unam.mx/index.php/2021/04/08/analisis-del-panorama-de-la-salud-en-la-frontera-norte-de-mexico/ (Accessed 12 January 2024).

Ruckert, A. *et al.* (2016) 'Global health diplomacy: a critical review of the literature', *Social Science & Medicine*, 55, pp. 61–72.

Scholten, P.W.A. (2013) 'Agenda dynamics and the multi-level governance of intractable policy controversies: the case of migrant integration policies in the Netherlands', *Policy Science*, 46, pp. 217–236.

Scholten, P.W.A. and Penninx, R. (2016) 'The multilevel governance of migration and integration', in Garcès-Mascarenãs, B. and Penninx, R. (eds.) *Integration processes and policies in Europe*. Heidelberg: Springer, pp. 91–108.

Stoeva, P. (2020) 'Dimensions of health security–a conceptual analysis', *Global Challenges*, 4(10), pp. 1–12.

U.S. Department of Health & Human Services (HHS) (2021) 'U.S.-Mexico border health commission activities', 12 July. [Online]. Available at: www.hhs.gov/about/agencies/oga/about-oga/what-we-do/international-relations-division/americas/border-health-commission/activities/index.html (Accessed 12 January 2024).

Valle, V.M. (2014) 'Private sector activities to reach millennium development goal six on the U.S.-Mexico border', *Voices of Mexico*, 98, pp. 98–105.

Vearey, J., Gruchy, T.D. and Maple, N. (2021) 'Global health (security), immigration governance and COVID-19 in South(ern) Africa: an evolving research agenda', *Journal of Migration and Health*, 3, pp. 1–8.

Velasco, J.L. (2014) 'U.S.-Mexico border health commission initiatives and activities', *Voices of Mexico*, 98, pp. 82–87. [Online]. Available at: www.revistascisan.unam.mx/Voices/no98.php (Accessed 12 January 2024).

World Health Organization (WHO) (2018) *Medicines, vaccines and health products access to medicines and vaccines. Report by the director-general*. [Online]. Available at: https://apps.who.int/gb/ebwha/pdf_files/EB144/B144_17-en.pdf (Accessed 12 January 2024).

6 Health Systems Resilience and the COVID-19 Pandemic in Ecuador and Mexico

María Gabriela Palacio Ludeña and Ricardo Velázquez Leyer

Introduction

The COVID-19 pandemic highlighted the urgency of building resilient public health systems. The concept of global health security (GHS) and health systems resilience came to the forefront of public debates with the pandemic that began in the first quarter of 2020. GHS was introduced by the World Health Organization (WHO) to set guidelines for the measures that national governments should adopt to prepare for health shocks. The development of resilient healthcare systems was one of the core recommendations of the GHS normative framework. This chapter compares the level of resilience of the Ecuadorean and Mexican healthcare systems to examine how well they were prepared for a health crisis like the pandemic and how the first actions to respond to it unfolded, to contribute to the literature on national healthcare provision and global health policy.

Ecuador and Mexico are chosen as typical case studies of the Latin American region because, despite exhibiting important differences, they share significant similarities in terms of healthcare concerning institutional and provision configurations and modes of fragmentation. These cases can shed light on the key factors determining the responsive capacity of healthcare systems in the region and the challenges faced in terms of safeguarding adequate levels of protection and mobilising resources at the national and international levels. Healthcare provisions in both countries consist of Bismarckian social insurance programmes with an additional layer for people not covered by social insurance and a considerable role played by private providers, representing the most common types of healthcare organisations in the region. Like various other Latin American countries, these are two countries that have been devastated by the pandemic; at the beginning of 2022, Ecuador registered 194 deaths per 100,000 people, the eighth highest in Latin America, and Mexico 234 COVID-19 crisis deaths per 100,000 people, the sixth highest rate in the region (WHO, 2022). These cases thus evince the strain placed on typical Latin American healthcare systems and the consequences of the pandemic.

DOI: 10.4324/9781003494959-6

The comparative analysis of the two cases is based on the analytical framework of health systems resilience proposed by Thomas *et al.* (2020). The framework is made up of 13 strategies that governments should undertake to strengthen the resilience of their healthcare systems. Since at the moment of writing of this chapter, the pandemic was still unfolding and it was not clear yet what would be the results in many areas, the chapter centres on the analysis of the seven strategies that, according to the framework, should have been in place when the pandemic began, as part of the preparation of a healthcare system against any shock.

Our analysis is based on both quantitative and qualitative evidence drawn from national and international official sources, reports by non-governmental organisations, and academic literature. We aim to provide a comprehensive understanding of the actions undertaken in each of the strategies in order to inform our findings about the contradictions and lack of coordination of global policy. Our conclusions highlight the political processes that shape government responses to pandemics. We anchor our analysis on pandemic politics, as the possibility of building a resilient health system is a result of the actions and inactions of various international and domestic political actors who interact across multiple levels. We show how the actions of some international organisations may act against the building up of resilient health systems and how the Ecuadorean and Mexican cases can illustrate developments that unfold in all five areas of pandemic politics presented in the introduction of this volume, namely, symbolic politics, disease diplomacy, compliance with international regulations, medical populism and the political economy of disease.

The rest of the chapter is organised as follows. The following section presents the analytical framework of health systems resilience and justifies its application for the research. The second part describes the Mexican and Ecuadorean healthcare systems, including an overview of recent developments. Next, we analyse the actions undertaken for the seven strategies in both cases and compare their results. The final segment compares the findings of each case and offers some concluding remarks.

Global Health Security and Health Systems Resilience

The concept of GHS is defined by the WHO as the actions required to minimise the effects of acute health emergencies that endanger people's health across regions and international borders (WHO, 2021). The topic acquired a top priority in the early 2000s, given the imminent risk of the spread of zoonotic diseases among humans in a scenario of wasteful consumption and travel, the threat of biological terrorism, but mostly the consequences of the loss of biodiversity and ecosystem integrity. As a result, the WHO modified its International Health Regulations (IHR) in 2005, which established the rules to face acute health emergencies that may spread internationally or might require a coordinated international response. The 2005

IHR expanded the scope of activities that member states should undertake to detect and contain diseases at local levels, assess and alert the global community of disease threats, and prevent and control contagions (Rodier *et al.*, 2007; WHO, 2021).[1] Annex 1 of the IHR described the core capacity requirements of national health infrastructure to detect, report, and control health emergencies of international concern, but without mentioning links to any optimal organisation of healthcare services to address such events (WHO, 2021).

An additional resolution was issued in 2011 to establish guidelines for strengthening the capacity of health systems to address health emergencies (WHO, 2011). The resolution mandated member states to protect investment in health infrastructure and strengthen the resilience of health systems; to integrate health emergency management programmes into national health plans; to develop and prepare hospital infrastructure to respond to internal and external emergencies; and to strengthen local health workforces through enhanced planning, training, and access to adequate resources (WHO, 2011). Yet, this resolution still did not specify concrete measures that governments should adopt to deal with acute health emergencies.

The WHO monitors compliance with IHR with an annual self-assessment carried out by each country and voluntary external evaluations conducted every four to five years. According to this framework, in 2017, the implementation status of IHR core capacities for Ecuador was 90% and for Mexico 95%. The adequacy of this framework to assess the capacity of a country to address health crises should be questioned, since a large majority of countries registered high implementation percentages of IHR core capacities like these two countries but were subsequently harshly affected by the COVID-19 pandemic. Moreover, only one category relates to the actual provision of healthcare (WHO, 2021). A Global Health Security Index was published by the Johns Hopkins Center for Health Security and two other organisations to assess compliance with the IHR (GHS, 2021), with information for 195 countries but only one category related to healthcare provision. Hence, Thomas *et al.* (2020) may represent a more comprehensive framework to assess countries' capacity to face health shocks.

The concept of health systems resilience encompasses the set of actions that governments should undertake to prepare their populations against the growing risk of acute health events (Thomas *et al.*, 2020). In their policy brief endorsed by the WHO, Thomas *et al.* (2020) specifically define resilience as the ability to prepare for, manage, and learn from health shocks, in turn defined as sudden and extreme changes that impact health systems, like pandemics, economic crises, or political conflicts. This contrasts with the predictable and common emphasis on demographic or epidemiological transitions. The authors conceptualised a shock as consisting of four stages that form a cycle: preparedness to shocks, shock onset and alert, shock impact and management, and recovery and learning. They identified 13 strategies that are required to enhance resilience during the four stages, classified according to the healthcare functions of governance, financing, resources, and service delivery to which they belonged (see Table 6.1).

The recommended governance strategies to have in place at the preparedness stage are effective and participatory leadership capable of preventing, detecting, and effectively addressing a public health threat with transparent communication, for which the building of trust and support and the existence of a legal mandate are fundamental characteristics; coordination of activities by relevant actors, which refers to the effective collaboration across sectors, state and civil society actors, as well as other governments and international organisations, to develop and implement adequate plans against health shocks; and effective information systems and flows, sharing critical information among stakeholders through functional communication channels involving hard infrastructure as well as the existence of freedoms of press and speech and the development of efficient surveillance systems.

For the financing function, the strategies for the preparedness stage are sufficient allocation and flexibility of monetary resources to ensure that the health budget is sufficient to meet demands and that it can be adjusted to face a health crisis; and comprehensive health coverage, with a generous package of services provided equally to the entire population, without which it will be challenging to adapt healthcare provision when a shock impacts the country.

Finally, the preparedness strategies for the resources function are the appropriate level and distribution of human and physical resources, like doctors, nurses, and other healthcare personnel, as well as hospitals and hospital beds, with the capacity of increasing them in case of a crisis; and a motivated and well-supported workforce in the resources function, who are found at the front line of the responses to health crises and are the most vulnerable in disease outbreaks.

The Ecuadorean and Mexican Healthcare Systems

This section discusses the healthcare systems in Ecuador and Mexico at the beginning of 2020. These two countries have been selected as they have similar healthcare systems, despite having different political systems and regimes, varying sizes, models, and levels of economic development. Both countries have healthcare systems of intermediate development among Latin American countries, established on Bismarckian principles with additional layers added later for people not covered by social insurance programmes. The private sector also plays a significant role in both countries. This analysis aims to identify the capacity and capabilities of healthcare provisioning to handle emergencies, especially those posed by the COVID-19 pandemic. We first provide a brief historical trajectory of both the Ecuadorian and Mexican systems to understand each respective state's ability to govern, manage, and deal with a crisis, following the approach of Mazzucato and Kattel (2020).

Table 6.1 Strategies to strengthen health system resilience

Function	Shock stage			
	Preparedness	Onset and alert	Impact and management	Recovery and learning
Governance	Effective and participatory leadership Coordination of activities across government and key stakeholders Effective information systems and flow	Organisational leaning culture that is responsive to crises Surveillance enabling timely detection of shocks and their impact		
Financing	Ensuring sufficient monetary resources in the system and flexibility to reallocate and inject extra funds Comprehensive health coverage	Ensuring stability of health system funding through countercyclical health financing mechanisms and reserves Purchasing flexibility of reallocation of funding to meet changing needs		
Resources	Appropriate level and distribution of human and physical resources Motivated and well supported workforce	Ability to increase capacity to cope with sudden surge in demand		
Service delivery		Alternative and flexible approaches to deliver care		

Source: Thomas et al. (2020)

The Ecuadorean System

Ecuador's public health system was initially established through the Social Security Medical Services in 1935 as part of the National Security System. It took several decades for the Ministry of Health to be created in 1967, during the state-led industrialisation period. This was done following the National Assembly's mandate to create a new constitution after three years of military dictatorship. At the time of its creation, Ecuador was the only country in Latin America without a Ministry of Health.

The Ministry of Health was created to provide universal coverage to the population. By 1970, it had completed its nationwide social infrastructure and became the primary supplier of health services to the Ecuadorian population, including remote rural areas. In 1970, the Direction for Health Promotion and Integral Health Attention was established, which oversaw coordinating attention, prevention, and promotion programmes.

In 1997, the Special Law for State Decentralization and Local Participation was introduced, delegating functions, powers, responsibilities, and resources, including financial ones, to municipalities to plan, coordinate, implement, and evaluate integral health programmes. However, most of the attention is still provided through the MSP network (47% of the medical units in the country) and the IESS network (10%).

In 1998, the health system was decentralised. Section 4, Article 45, of the 1998 constitution indicates that the state will organise a healthcare system that integrates all public, autonomous, private, and communal entities of the sector. However, due to administrative and political reasons, this decentralisation was not fully implemented, and the MSP (or Ministry of Public Health) kept its role as the main health provider. In the latest constitution of 2008, there was no mention of decentralisation in health (Goldman, 2009).

At the central government level, the MSP regulates health promotion through the National Directorate of Promotion and Integral Attention (OEA, 2016). The Public Health Ministry encompasses about 1,340 organisations, foundations, and associations directly involved in health promotion. Their participation is regulated by the Executive Decree No. 656 of April 13, 2015, as governed by the Sectoral Citizen Health Council (Lucio, Villacrés and Henríquez, 2011).

The healthcare system is organised into seven subsystems that add up to the Integral Network of Public Healthcare, or Red Pública Integral de Salud (RPIS): state-MEF-MSP (60.63%), IESS-SGSFI (23.20%), MIDENA-ISS-FA (0.87%), MDI-ISSPOL (0.85%), MDTOP-ANT-SPRAT (n/a), and a private for and non-profit (9%). These subsystems supply different packages to the populations they serve, under either the affiliate's or citizen/beneficiary's logic. Health services are provided through their network, across networks (since 2012), or by external parties working under the Complementary Network or Red Complementaria (RC), which are later compensated for providing health services. The RPIS, together with private providers, serves 90% of the Ecuadorian population. The private sector coverage is hard to estimate, as people in the highest income groups are usually under-represented in the household surveys used to calculate health coverage (Lucio, Villacrés and Henríquez, 2011). In practice, the system is fragmented, as not all private providers collaborate with the public healthcare network. Doctors tend to be concentrated in big cities, which adds a layer of spatial segregation to the already uneven access to healthcare.

Coverage is highly segregated according to occupational status, which determines the levels of entitlements and provision schemes. Though the 2008 constitution explicitly states the state as a guarantor of universal insurance, there is no insurance scheme available to all citizens. The general social security scheme, IESS, provides entitlements to registered workers in formal employment, self-employed workers (autonomous), business owners, and non-remunerated family workers. Other insurance schemes, such as ISSPOL, cover the police and ISSFA, the army. The Farmers' Social Security (Seguro Social Campesino—created in 1968 and subsidised by the state) grants independent workers in agriculture and fisheries entitlements in terms of access to health, disability, and old-age pensions, thus serving rural populations. A Beveridge scheme based on taxes, for example, tax income and VAT, complements the System of Universal Insurance (Sistema de Aseguramiento Universal) based on contributions (Bismarck).

The Mexican System

At the beginning of 2020, the public system was made up of separate layers that offered coverage to different population groups, depending on the occupational status of the household's breadwinner. Several social insurance agencies provided coverage to different categories of formal sector workers; the two largest were the Mexican Social Insurance Institute (IMSS), which covered private sector employees, and the Social Security and Services Institute for State Workers (ISSSTE), which covered federal civil servants, plus special schemes for workers of the state oil company, the military, and employees of state governments. Social insurance agencies acted as both health insurers and providers of primary, secondary, and tertiary health services, funded by contributions from workers, employers, and the state. Each agency operated separately, with its own legal framework, administration, human resources, and infrastructure (González Block *et al.*, 2020).

For people not covered by social insurance, the creation of the National Institute for Health Welfare (INSABI) was meant to provide healthcare as a citizenship right. This population group is large for two reasons: the legal exclusion from IMSS mandatory social insurance of anyone without a formal employment relation, for example, the self-employed or employers, and because of widespread evasion of that mandatory insurance by employers and employees. In early 2020, INSABI had just been launched to replace a health insurance programme that offered healthcare to the same population group targeted by INSABI, albeit on a voluntary basis and with the payment of contributions, although low-income families, which constituted the majority of the insured population, were exempt. Like social insurance schemes, INSABI functioned as a separate government agency that operated services with its own resources and infrastructure but was funded with general taxes and began operations only covering primary and secondary services (INSABI, 2020; Reich, 2020).

The private sector also plays a large role in the provision of healthcare services. Private services have mostly operated independently from public services with low levels of government regulation. In early 2020, public social insurance schemes could subcontract private services when their supply could not meet the demand for an intervention, and under IMSS legislation, the payment of health insurance contributions could be discounted if employers supplied healthcare services to their employees, but these options were scantly applied, and in fact the use of the second one had been in decline in recent years. Hence, the private healthcare sector has operated under a market supply and demand rationale, providing a wide range of services from primary care to highly specialised tertiary care. The deficient supply of public services across all schemes, worse in the case of services for people without social insurance coverage, explains the large role of the private sector; the poor quality and limited access of public programmes implicitly incentivises or forces many people of all income levels to use private services,[2] but with a difference in the type of service. Low-income people could only access private primary care, while interventions that require hospitalisations are only affordable to high-income groups (González Block *et al.*, 2018, 2020).

The federal Secretariat for Health (SS) is responsible for emitting public health measures and regulations of public and private healthcare provision. Each state also has a health secretariat, which coordinates the application of federal legislation in its jurisdiction. Until 2019, states' health secretariats were also responsible for administering the healthcare services offered by the Popular Health Insurance to people with no social insurance; from early 2020, INSABI sought to centralise those services, although several state governments did not sign the agreements to give up their services (Reich, 2020).

The General Health Council (CGS) represents another tier of public authority on health matters. This council is a collegiate body that is a direct dependency of the Presidency of the Republic, is presided over by the federal Health Secretary, and is integrated by the heads of several federal government departments and academic and professional institutions. The approval and publication of the declaration of health emergencies, as well as their management, are among the core responsibilities assigned to this body in the legislation. An executive board integrated by the Health Secretary, the IMSS and ISSSTE directors, as well as any other member designated by the president, has the responsibility of managing the cases of health emergencies (IGHS, 2021).

Strategies for Healthcare Resilience in Ecuador and Mexico

This section compares the strategies adopted in each country for preparedness against health shocks, according to the analytical framework proposed by Thomas *et al.* (2020). Seven strategies are analysed, belonging to the healthcare functions of governance, financing, and resources. The analysis covers the unfolding of each strategy up to and during the pandemic. We are particularly interested in discussing the health sector's capacity to perform emergency responses during policy design and implementation, thus the emphasis on aspects of governance (including effective and participatory leadership).

Resilience Strategies in Ecuador

Once the pandemic's epicentre moved to the region, Ecuador was soon identified as one of the countries hardest hit globally, next to Peru (*Financial Times*, 2020a). Nevertheless, the actual mortality is likely to be under-represented due to the scarcity of tests, the additional deaths from treatable diseases resulting from the limited access to intensive care units (ICUs), and the general collapse of the health sector in Ecuador. Various estimates of excess mortality in Ecuador, that is, the number of deaths above the historical average for a specific period as recorded in civil registries, show that the number of fatalities was higher than those reported by the government. In the middle of an infodemic, deferred responses, political fragmentation, fiscal constraints, and growing polarisation, Ecuador became an early global symbol of the devastating effects of COVID-19 (King *et al.*, 2020).

Effective and Participatory Leadership

On March 12, 2020, the government decreed an emergency in all health centres in the country affiliated with the National Health System, including laboratory facilities, units of epidemiology and control, air ambulances, medical and paramedical services, hospitalisation, and outpatient clinics. This Ministerial Decree directly responded to the imminent effects of the COVID-19 virus and aimed at preventing an outbreak. Following the declaration of COVID-19 as a global pandemic by the WHO on March 16, 2020, the government decreed a state of exception, given the exponential growth in the number of confirmed cases. The state of exception in practice meant limited mobility, that is, the freedom to transit and the right to free association and reunion, a strict restriction imposed to guarantee the observance of social distancing and quarantine measures. It also declared a curfew on March 17, 2020, while designating exempted groups whose mobility was permitted to assist in the public response to the pandemic, namely the National Police, Armed Forces, and health personnel. Thus, the state of emergency declaration was deemed necessary to coordinate the public response, mobilise the state's resources, and prioritise public expenditure. However, there was weak coordination with subnational governments because of either inaccurate or incomplete data (Plan-V, 2020), poor enforcement of sanctions (El Comercio, 2020c), and a lack of harmonisation of policies and responses with municipalities (El Comercio, 2020a).

There was harsh criticism against the central and local governments for the noticeable lack of coordination. The first confirmed COVID-19 case was reported on February 29, 2020. Within a few weeks, and with a population of over two million inhabitants, the city of Guayaquil became the first COVID-19 hotspot. The government struggled to bury the dead while bodies were left in the streets of Guayaquil—not all attributable to the virus as tests were not widely available. A combination of collective panic, misinformation, and the collapse of burial services led to jarring images that made Ecuador infamous in global news outlets. By late March, the Municipal Director of Hygiene and Markets of the city announced the necessity to prepare a mass grave to bury about 300 bodies in Guayaquil (BBC, 2020), further exacerbating collective panic and discontent with the government's response.

Coordination with and among local governments was particularly challenging. Municipalities had a high level of independence regarding the type and strictness of containment measures. Tensions between the central and local governments resulted in a geographically differentiated and uncoordinated response. To diminish discretional local responses, by early 2022, the central government, via the Committee for Emergency Operation (Comité de Operaciones de Emergencias, or COE), intervened and regulated the risk responses by creating a dashboard (Semáforo de Protección de COVID-19) that alerted the public of the level of cases per municipality and province and standardised the measures to be adopted according to the severity of the situation.

Coordination of Activities Across Government and Key Stakeholders

During the first weeks of the pandemic, there was weak coordination with subnational governments, either because of inaccurate or incomplete data (Plan-V, 2020), inadequate enforcement of sanctions (El Comercio, 2020c), or a lack of harmonisation of policies and responses among municipalities (El Comercio, 2020a). For instance, municipalities could determine the level of alertness in their territories and adopt containment measures such as lockdowns, depending on the perceived severity of the COVID-19 cases and estimated health response capacity. This resulted in ambiguities in risk assessment, with municipalities shifting the alert codes discretionally.

Regarding coordination with key international actors, before the pandemic, Ecuador had adopted the Cooperation Strategy 2018–2022, which determined the priorities of technical cooperation between the WHO and the Ecuadorian government to contribute to the objectives of the Development Plan 2017–2021 and the Sustainable Health Agenda for the Americas 2018–2030 (ASSA). Among the areas of cooperation, the emphasis was on strengthening the National Health System to achieve universal access to health, the application of IHR, and attention to early mortality for chronic diseases and attention to vulnerable groups following a rights-based logic (intercultural and gender awareness).

During the pandemic, the WHO office in Ecuador coordinated with the Ecuadorian government and other organisations, such as UNICEF, UNDP, CARE, and the Red Cross, among others, to establish basic technical norms. Among these, it is worth mentioning the Protocol for Intercultural Awareness for the Prevention and Attention of COVID-19 for Peoples and Indigenous Nations, Afro Ecuadorians, and Montubios in Ecuador (Protocolo con Pertinencia Intercultural para la Prevención y Atención de la COVID-19 en Pueblos y Nacionalidades Indígenas, Afroecuatorianos y Montubios del Ecuador) (Consejo Nacional para la Igualdad de Pueblos y Nacionalidades, 2020). It was implemented to approach community leaders to coordinate actions with public entities, particularly humanitarian aid and transport. Next to this, the Confederation of Indigenous Nations of Ecuador (Confederación de Nacionalidades Indígenas del Ecuador, or CONAIE) and the Confederation of Indigenous Nationalities of the Ecuadorian Amazon (Confederación de Nacionalidades Indígenas de la Amazonía Ecuatoriana, or CONFENIAE) adopted voluntary measures, such as self-quarantine within peoples and indigenous nations' territories and prohibiting activities such as tourism (Altmann *et al.*, 2020).

Effective Information Systems and Flow

Public information campaigns and protocols for the attention of vulnerable populations were set in motion in Ecuador during the pandemic. Nevertheless, according to a study by the Central University of Ecuador, only 39% of the population reported knowing the reasons why quarantine measures were set in place in the country (Altmann *et al.*, 2020). Also, as was the case in many other countries, there was controversy regarding the actual number of deaths attributed to the pandemic. While Sebastián Naranjo (2020), senior analyst at Cálculo Electoral, a data analysis group, reports a level 230% higher than the usual figures for April 2020—equivalent to 14,460 deaths—a *New York Times* Big Data analysis estimates that the mortality in Ecuador was 15 times higher than the official number of COVID-19 deaths reported by the government for the same period (*New York Times*, 2020). As of December 2020, Naranjo estimates a total excess mortality of 37,753, considering civil registry data for the period March 12 to December 17, 2020, when compared to historical averages for these months in 2017, 2018, and 2019, as obtained from the Statistics Department, INEC, and published by the Civil Registry (Registro Social). Yet Ortiz-Pardo and Fernández-Naranjo argue that these estimates, based on historical weekly or monthly mean values, were sensible to outliers and thus misleading. During the first phases of the pandemic, the country suffered from an "infodemic," for the ambiguity in the numbers led to either alarmist and politicised responses or aloofness and delayed responses.

Other intersecting issues started to surface as the pandemic progressed and information reached media outlets and civil society organisations. On March 27, the Committee for National Emergencies (Comité de Operaciones de Emergencia Nacional, or COE) released the Protocol for the Communication and Attention of Gender and Intrafamilial Violence during the COVID-19 Emergency (Protocolo de Comunicación y Atención de Casos de Violencia de Género e Intrafamiliar en la Emergencia por Coronavirus (COVID-19)) (COE, 2020). This protocol was drafted in response to the plea of women's rights activists who had highlighted the increase in gender violence, following the recommendation of the Follow-up Mechanism to the Belém do Pará Convention (or MESECVI) of the Organization for the American States (OAS). On March 31, the National Council for the Equality of Disabilities (Consejo Nacional para la Igualdad de Discapacidades, or CONADIS) (CONADIS, 2020) released a protocol for persons with disabilities and their families: Guide for the Prevention and Attention for the COVID-19 Exposure of People with Disability and in a Condition of Temporal Disability, and Their Families (Guía de prevención y atención por contagio del virus COVID-19 en personas con discapacidad y en condición discapacitante temporal y sus familias), which offers general guidelines to prevent the spread of COVID-19 while caring for persons with permanent or temporary disabilities, both at home and in the community, in particular, norms regarding hygiene and psychological health.

Ensuring Sufficient Monetary Resources in the System and Flexibility to Reallocate and Inject Extra Funds

The Ecuadorean healthcare system, due to limited fiscal capacity, had run large deficits and suffered from underinvestment, with shortages of workers prior to the pandemic. As of 2019, there was a deficit of about US$3,655 billion (approximately 3.2% of GDP), according to Lucio *et al.* (2019). Domestic private health expenditure as a percentage of current health expenditure was 48%. Furthermore, the health system is vulnerable to shocks, given that the financing is heavily reliant on either formal sector contributions (which are pro-cyclical and limited given the high levels of informality) or the central budget, which poses evident liquidity constraints dependent on the business cycle, including the capacity of workers to contribute to the system through taxes and contributions and the reliance of government revenues on extractive rent.

The cutbacks in public healthcare expenditure were exacerbated by the International Monetary Fund's (IMF's) call for fiscal adjustment within the framework of the Extended Arrangement Under the Extended Fund Facility of 2019 (Naciones Unidas, 2020), including a significant layoff of public healthcare workers who could have supported the health response during the pandemic (Naciones Unidas, 2020). However, the IMF provided funding to support the country's stabilisation and recovery programme: a US$6.5 billion Extended Fund Facility arrangement on September 30, 2020. The new Extended Fund Facility of December 15, 2020, called for further fiscal adjustment equal to 5.5% of the gross domestic product (Progressive International, 2020). While the government failed to make US$200 million in bond interest payments due to the health crisis, it still made a US$325 million principal payment on its sovereign bonds due in March 2020 (*Financial Times*, 2020b) and reached an agreement with its bondholders on August 3, 2020 to restructure its US$17.4 billion of sovereign debt (*Financial Times*, 2020c). The government had to navigate these external pressures in the face of strong opposition for prioritising debt servicing (CDES, 2020) and the possibility of significant social and political unrest—as alerted by mobilisations amid the restrictions in October 2020 (El Comercio, 2020b), echoing the 12 days of protests in October 2019 that followed the announcement of the end to a fuel subsidy and a series of austerity reforms recommended by the IMF as part of a plan to reduce public debt (Díaz Pabón and Palacio Ludeña, 2021). These external constraints further limited the public health response to the COVID-19 pandemic.

Universal Health Coverage

Access to the public healthcare system, as provided by the Health Ministry, or MSP, is based on both (registered) residency and citizenship. Yet, the actual capacity is limited. Most comprehensive health services are accessible only to those affiliated with the branches' social security systems: IESS, ISSFA, and ISSPOL (Lucio, Villacrés and Henríquez, 2011) or via private providers, as shown in Table 6.2.

Financing is organised through the National Health System, in which funding comes from taxes and state royalties (central budget) and is executed through fiscal transfers. Next to this, the National Insurance System is financed through social security (IESS, ISSFA, and ISSPOL) contributions. The system has been increasingly commodified, as health funding is increasingly channelled to the private sector. There are significant barriers to accessing health services. A significant share of the population is not affiliated with the social

Table 6.2 Healthcare coverage indicators of Ecuador

Percentage of population covered by government schemes and private schemes	12.2%
Percentage of population covered by social insurance schemes	IESS: 29.2%
Percentage of population uncovered	58.6%

Source: INEC (2019)

security systems, which results in staggering differences between different sectors, formal and informal. This results in non-covered populations resorting to private providers, when available, with ruinous out-of-pocket expenses. For example, in 2018, the out-of-pocket payments as a percentage of current health expenditure were 40% (WHO, 2021). With the public healthcare system overloaded with COVID-19 patients, many low- and middle-income and informal populations were left to their own means to secure access to health services, with an increase in the co-morbidity due to a lack of timely attention to otherwise treatable diseases.

Appropriate Level and Distribution of Human and Physical Resources

As of 2020, for every 10,000 people, the number/density of doctors was 23.44 and for nurses, 14.54 (as reported for 2018), while the number/density of beds in public, for-profit, and not-for-profit institutions was 741 surgery rooms, 369 delivery rooms, 205 ICUs, and 204 intermediate care rooms, also for 2018 (OIT, 2021). The system was evidently understaffed. According to an ILO study, in November 2020, the public healthcare system had only managed to provide medical attention to 60% of the patients covered during 2019, with the most significant reduction taking place in IESS-related hospitals, approximately 39% (OIT, 2021). There has been a significant effort to make use of virtual medical visits and expand remote outpatient care to serve the most vulnerable populations (those aged 60 and above). Furthermore, from the 4,165 in- and out-patient health centres, both public and private, only 626 could provide in-patient care (about 15%) (Observatorio Social, 2020). This means that even if these centres could diagnose COVID-19 cases, they did not have the capacity to hospitalise them, and among the latter, very few centres had an ICU.

In addition, these figures do not even consider the territorial and urban-rural divides, which played a role in the unequal distribution of COVID-19-related deaths, correlated to the unequal provision of human and physical resources across the country. Not only financial but also geographical barriers have impeded access to prevention, testing, and treatment of illness, particularly evident during the pandemic. The three largest provinces, Guayas, Pichincha, and Manabí, concentrate nearly 40% of the total health centres in the country, next to provinces in the Amazon region and Galapagos Islands that have a low density of health centres relative to the population. However, these provinces have the highest proportion of healthcare professionals relative to the total population, for example, Pastaza: 57 doctors and nurses per 1,000 inhabitants, indicating a mismatch between physical and human resources.

Motivated and Well-Supported Workforce

Emergency responses to deal with the pandemic in the context of limited resources resulted in a reduced ability to respond to other illnesses and conditions. With health workers overworked and underpaid, the risk that exposure to viruses and other contaminants translated into fatalities among critical staff increased dramatically. It is estimated that between 2019 and 2020, nearly 3,000 (public) healthcare workers were fired and about 2,279 were made redundant during the pandemic (Palacio Ludeña, 2023). In addition, it should be noted that until late 2019, Cuba had been an important international actor in the health sector, under a bilateral cooperation framework that allowed for Cuban doctors' participation in health provisioning in the country. Though the central government introduced a series of incentives, both financial and non-financial, many hospitals were understaffed due to the continued cuts in personnel.

There was also an imbalance in terms of the proportion of doctors and nurses per medical establishment, resulting in the possibility of diagnosing COVID-19 cases but having to refer patients to other centres that had enough personnel.

Resilience Strategies in Mexico

Effective and Participatory Leadership

Mexico has been one of the countries most affected by the pandemic. The number of cases that are reported in official statistics results from the low levels of testing, much lower than in any comparable country. The real impact of the pandemic is revealed by other indicators, like the excess mortality rate from all causes of 55% during 2020 and the first semester of 2021 (OECD, 2021).

The leadership role in the government's response to the pandemic was assigned by the president to the office of the Undersecretary for Health Prevention and Promotion (UHPP). The CGS, established in the legislation as a collegiate body with a mandate to act and emit policies and rules in cases of health emergencies, has played only a minor or even insignificant role. The CGS was not summoned for the first time until March 19, more than one month after the WHO had declared the coronavirus outbreak a public health emergency of international concern, and it did not declare a health emergency due to COVID-19 until March 30. Even the Health Secretary played a secondary role to the Undersecretary. The outcome of the type of leadership that has been exerted has been the excessive centralisation and politicisation of decision-making, with dire consequences for the fight against the pandemic (IGHS, 2021).

The decision taken by the president to delegate authority to the UHPP could be understood as the need to optimise the management of the pandemic, but far from achieving that aim, it caused a number of problems that undermined the government's response. The centralisation of authority in a small department of the federal government obstructed the development of public deliberation and learning processes, crucial to formulating, adapting, and implementing public policy in a challenging and dynamic environment like the one created by the pandemic.[3]

When the pandemic struck, the country was already experiencing unprecedented levels of political polarisation due to constant public attacks by President López Obrador against any actor who disagreed with the orientation of his policies. The head of the UHPP, Hugo López-Gatell Ramírez, who personally assumed the protagonist role, frequently put the blame on the pandemic and its impacts on other social and political actors, attacking anyone who questioned the government's decisions, creating recurrent political frictions that obstructed collaboration with other government levels and departments.

As a result of the type of leadership that was generated, decisions were made on political grounds and not on a technical basis, ignoring advice offered by various international and domestic governments, as well as academic and professional organisations.[4] For example, no massive testing programme or serious contact tracing was ever introduced, and the federal government refused to recommend or mandate the use of masks.

Coordination of Activities Across Government and Key Stakeholders

The centralisation and politicisation of the federal government's pandemic response impeded the coordination with other government and non-government actors, which was fundamental to ameliorating the pandemic's negative effects. Notwithstanding the complexity of coordinating a response to a health emergency in a federal system of government, the leadership style displayed by the UHPP generated recurrent quarrels with other state actors. State and municipal governments were not considered for the formulation of the measures to face the crises, nor were they included in their implementation. For example, the traffic light system was designed without the participation of subnational governments, prompting many state governments to ignore or create their own monitoring systems (IGHS, 2021).

Coordination with other federal healthcare agencies, like IMSS and ISSSTE, seemed to have been close, which could have been expected as they are also under the direct authority of the president. Nonetheless, advice and suggestions to combat the pandemic from academia, civil society, or Congress were not only ignored, but their proponents were also labelled political adversaries and attacked on a political basis. The neglect of the CGS eliminated a space where adequate coordination could have been achieved and valuable knowledge to improve the response could have been exchanged (IGHS, 2021).

The private health sector was possibly the only non-governmental stakeholder with whom a relatively successful coordination was developed. Agreements were made early on to treat beneficiaries of public health insurance schemes in private hospitals, but they covered only seven interventions (SS, 2020).[5] Moreover, the federal government showed contempt for private providers when it refused to include many private health personnel in the first vaccination campaigns (IGHS, 2021), with dire consequences for these employees.

Effective Information Systems and Flow

Since 2006, the prevalence of respiratory illnesses has been monitored through a sentinel system that collected information from a national representative sample of health centres and hospitals across the country. The system was employed to monitor the development of the COVID-19 pandemic, but the decision to reduce the number of units of the sample and the particular characteristics of the new virus rendered it useless. The large number of infected people with mild symptoms or who were asymptomatic and did not turn up at health facilities disabled the system's capacity to survey the evolution of the number and location of cases and deaths and to serve as an instrument to plan actions to respond to the pandemic. Suggestions from a wide variety of international and domestic actors to use massive testing as a more effective tool to measure the extension of this particular pandemic were ignored by the public officials in charge of the response (IGHS, 2021). The decision to use the system to project an epidemiological curve based on the data it produced and to reject the application of testing led to the initial and erroneous assertion by the government that the pandemic would be over by May 2020. Mexico would become one of the countries with the lowest number of tests performed per population in the world (IGHS, 2021; OECD, 2021).

The government organised daily press conferences to inform the public on the development of the pandemic, but rather than assuring transparency, they became politicised spaces where the Undersecretary for Health Promotion and Prevention constantly sought quarrels with actors who did not agree with his management of the crisis. He and other public officials usually employed an overtechnical language that impeded the clear communication of the pandemic and the government's actions to the public.

Ensuring Sufficient Monetary Resources in the System and Flexibility to Reallocate and Inject Extra Funds

The social insurance layers of the public healthcare system, namely, IMSS and ISSSTE, are funded by tripartite contributions by employees, employers, and the state. Until 2019, the layer for people with no social insurance, that is, SPS, was funded by contributions from insured families and individuals and earmarked contributions by the federal and state governments, including earmarked funds for catastrophic health expenses and tertiary medical care.

Public health spending levels peaked during the second decade of the present century due to the expansion of coverage through the SPS. In 2013, public spending reached 3.1% of GDP and 53.8% of total health spending, while in per capita terms, it peaked at US$565 in 2016. The growing trend was reversed in the second half of the decade; by 2019, the year before the pandemic, public spending represented 2.7% of GDP, 49.3% of total spending, and US$558 per capita (OECD, 2022). The reasons for these decreasing trends may be found in the fragmented healthcare architecture, which, after an initial boost to public spending due to the expansion of voluntary health insurance, obstructed the further aggregation of political preferences for a better supply of public services, along with the large role performed by the private sector, which reaches diverse population groups, including low-income families who can afford primary care in private doctors' offices, many times adjacent to pharmacies (Bernales-Baksai and Velázquez Leyer, 2021; González Block *et al.*, 2018).

The large role performed by the private sector reveals a strong dependence on market provision to meet healthcare needs in the country. Even if covered by a public scheme, many people choose or are forced to use private services because of the low quality of and limited access to public services. In fact, of the total number of people who reported frequent use of private services in 2013, 46% were covered by a public scheme, a proportion that increased to 60% in 2017 (INSP, 2021). Private services are mostly funded through out-of-pocket spending; in 2019, it represented 42% of total health spending (WHO, 2021).

The scarcity and precariousness of monetary resources did not improve in 2020. An increase in public spending to 3.1% of GDP is explained by the downfall in economic output caused by the pandemic, and while the government was able to inject additional funds into the system, they were mostly taken from the catastrophic health expenses fund that existed under the SPS, which the government appropriated since the new scheme for people without social insurance, INSABI, only covered primary and secondary care.

Universal Health Coverage

The public healthcare system has never reached the entire population. Public provision has consisted of different social insurance programmes for specific categories of labour market insiders, that is, formal sector employees and their families, and additional layers for people without social insurance coverage. By 2017, 82% of the population were insured by a public scheme, an expansion that represents a significant improvement compared to only 40% who were insured in 2000 but still left one-fifth of the population uncovered (INEGI, 2017). Moreover, that figure masks the process of implicit commodification that unfolds as many people, even if publicly insured, choose or are forced to seek treatment in the private sector due to deficiencies in the supply of public services (Bernales-Baksai and Velázquez Leyer, 2021). Hence, before the pandemic began, the country was still far from achieving universal health coverage, measured not only by the percentage of people who may have legal coverage but also by outputs and outcomes related to real access and generous and equitable provision of public services provided to the majority of the population (Martínez Franzoni and Sánchez Ancochea, 2016).

Instead of signalling progress towards universal coverage, the recent healthcare reform of 2020 represents a regression. The fragmentation and inequalities of the public system were reproduced and exacerbated since INSABI only replaced Popular Health Insurance. There was no attempt at unifying all public schemes. Tertiary care, which represents the main cause of catastrophic medical expenses that are unaffordable in the private sector for the majority of the population, was effectively excluded. No significant additional resources necessary to expand provision have been allocated in real terms, such that the healthcare budget for 2021 did not increase in relation to the 2020 budget, which considering the increase in demand due to the pandemic is also a step backwards. No plan for improving the quality and expanding social insurance services has been announced. Additionally, an attempt at reforming the medicines procurement system triggered serious supply disruptions and has only generated shortages across the country, especially of drugs needed to treat expensive diseases like various types of cancer (Reich, 2020).

The implicit commodification of healthcare intensified during the pandemic. Although the government expanded facilities for COVID-19 patients, the overwhelming demands left many patients suffering from other illnesses unprotected. Because of these unmet demands and the deficiencies of public schemes, especially the newly created INSABI, 56% of people who required medical care were treated in the private sector in 2020, and 45% and 57% of IMSS and ISSSTE beneficiaries preferred or were pushed to use private services. Among people who had COVID-19, only 14% were treated in public hospitals or clinics.[6] Only 29% of people take into consideration entitlement to a public scheme when deciding where to seek care; the rest consider other variables related to quality and access (INSP, 2021). These indicators reveal the challenges that the country still has to overcome in order to even get near an authentic type of universal healthcare provision.

Appropriate Level and Distribution of Human and Physical Resources

The levels of human resources have improved during the present century. The number of doctors per 1,000 population passed from 1.6 in 2000 to 2.4 in 2019 (OECD, 2021), and from that total, the proportion of doctors employed in the public sector increased from 59% in 2000 to 71% in 2016 (González Block *et al.*, 2018). During the same period, the number of nurses increased from 2.2 to 2.9 per 1,000 population (OECD, 2022), of which more than 90% are employed in the public sector (González Block *et al.*, 2018). These changes are explained by the expansion of public healthcare provision through the SPS (González Block, 2020). Nonetheless, despite improvements, these levels of human resources were still below OECD averages, which registered 3.3 doctors and 8.9 nurses per 1,000 people in 2018 (OECD, 2022).[7]

The improvements in levels of human resources have not been matched by those of physical resources. During the current century, the number of hospitals has only grown 0.3% (González Block *et al.*, 2020), while the number of hospital beds per 1,000 population decreased from 1.05 in 2000 to 0.97 (OECD, 2022). Of the total number of beds, 76% correspond to public hospitals (González Block *et al.*, 2020). Deep geographical inequalities are observed across the country in both human and physical resources. Poor and rural regions register a much lower supply. The uneven distribution of public and private resources reinforces health inequalities. For example, the rate of medical specialists per 1,000 people drops from more than 4 in the wealthy state of Nuevo León to 0.4 in the poorest state of Chiapas, while the number of public hospital beds per 100,000 people ranges from 177 in Mexico City to 43 in Chiapas (González Block, 2020).

Hospital capacity was expanded to face the pandemic. The federal government has argued that due to this measure, no COVID-19 patient was left untreated. Some degree of success can be claimed in that regard; however, three important points must be considered. First, many COVID-19 patients were sent back to their homes to avoid the saturation of hospitals, creating a high percentage of COVID-19-related deaths occurring at home, more than 50% of the total according to some estimates after the first year of the pandemic. Second, the differences in the quality of the supply of private and public services were made evident in the much lower mortality rates registered in the former than in the latter. Finally, the focus on COVID-19 left untreated many patients who suffered from other diseases, fuelling the high excess mortality rate of the country (IGHS, 2021).

Motivated and Well-Supported Workforce

Evidence exists of growing support for the healthcare workforce in recent years. The number of physicians that graduated from university increased by 2.3% annually between 2003 and 2017; the rate of specialists that were graduating as a proportion of the total population was higher than the OECD average. Nursing became a popular undergraduate programme, with an annual enrolment growth of 18.2% in the last decade. Lastly, the wage earnings of health workers are higher in the public sector than in the private sector (González Block *et al.*, 2018).

Diagnosed problems include the relative neglect of primary care and health promotion and prevention in training curricula and the lack of explicit and transparent standards for professionals in both the public and private sectors (González Block *et al.*, 2018). During the pandemic, medical personnel across the country protested insufficient levels of workforce support, including a lack of training and personal protective equipment (PPE). Constant reports were presented in the media of the inadequate supply of training and equipment provided by the federal government. One year after the pandemic began, 329 public demonstrations of this sort were reported. The neglect of the required support resulted in Mexico becoming the country with the highest mortality rate in the world among health workers in 2020, according to Amnesty International. The Pan-American Health Organization (PAHO) reported in February 2021 that, out of 17 countries in the Americas, Mexican health workers accounted for 45% of COVID-19 deaths among healthcare personnel (Agren, 2020, IGHS, 2021).

The Comparison of Strategies in Ecuador and Mexico

This comparison of the strategies adopted by the Ecuadorean and Mexican governments to prepare against health emergencies reveals similar weaknesses. Some improvements were achieved during the present century, but they were insufficient to build up the necessary resilience to face a health shock like the COVID-19 pandemic. As can be observed in Table 6.3, the existing institutional architecture was not effectively or efficiently activated

Table 6.3 Health shock preparedness in Ecuador and Mexico

Strategy	Ecuador	Mexico
Effective and participatory leadership	Delayed responses and a lack of effective leadership from the central government	Politicisation and centralisation of leadership by a reduced number of federal officials
Coordination of activities across government and key stakeholders	Lack of coordination with subnational governments and nongovernmental actors; late adoption of technical norms	Lack of coordination with subnational governments and nongovernmental actors
Effective information systems and flows	Deficient information flows and discretionary risk assessment at the local level	Deficient information flows due to a refusal to adopt massive testing
Ensuring sufficient monetary resources in the system and flexibility to reallocate and inject extra funds	Insufficient monetary resources and no flexibility due to external financial pressures and vulnerabilities to the business cycle	Insufficient availability of public monetary resources and high dependence on private spending
Comprehensive health coverage	A fragmented public system with reduced coverage levels and occupational and regional segregation	A fragmented public system with reduced coverage levels and an intensification of implicit commodification processes
Appropriate levels and distribution of human and physical resources	Unequal distribution of human and physical resources and unbalanced share of resources within territories	Unequal distribution of human and physical resources
Motivated and well-supported workforce	Limited support and further cuts in health personnel	Limited support provided to fight the pandemic

Source: Authors' own elaboration

to assure strong leadership and close and timely coordination between relevant political and social actors, while fragmented Bismarckian healthcare systems left large sectors of the populations unprotected and dependent on private provision, and the limited and unequal distribution of physical and human resources hampered the capacity to respond to the crises.

However, important differences can also be observed in the design and implementation of several strategies that stem from the particular domestic political economy arrangements of each case and their relation with global policy, as illustrated in Figure 6.1. In Ecuador, resilience was hampered by the challenges of keeping a resource-based economy afloat. COVID-19 has exposed the financial weaknesses of export-oriented and debt-dependent economies (Büscher *et al.*, 2021). Ecuador's President Lenin Moreno even referred to this period as "the real first world war" (*Financial Times*, 2020d). Despite efforts to put finances on a strong footing, the oil-dependent Ecuadorian economy was hamstrung financially. It grapples with US$58.4 billion of total debt, more than half its annual gross domestic product (*Financial Times*, 2020b). With energy prices at a historical minimum and damage to the country's two main oil pipelines (*Financial Times*, 2020d), as a dollarised economy, the only influence it has over the money supply is preventing outflows.

Ecuador's ability to make policy decisions has been limited primarily due to strict global governance rules. These rules have made it difficult to sustain investments in the healthcare sector, retain and expand skills and

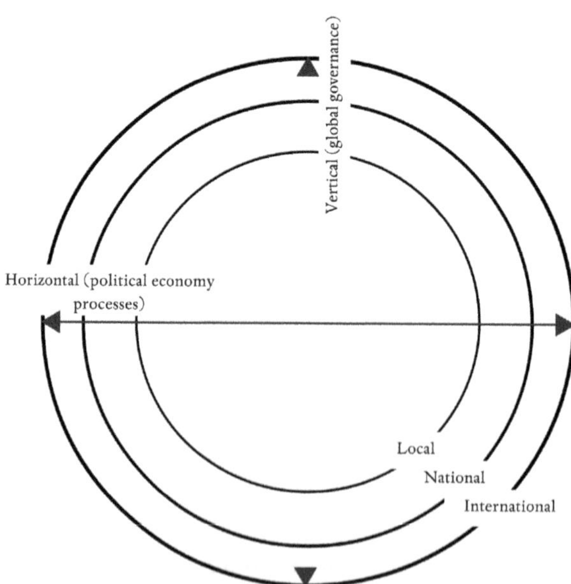

Figure 6.1 Global governance and horizontal political economy loops

capabilities within the public sector, and coordinate with private actors to tackle emergencies. The country's response to the COVID-19 pandemic was also hampered by financial constraints and international trade challenges, which resulted in delayed responses from the public sector during the crisis and its aftermath. While emergency cash transfers were provided as part of the social protection response, the country struggled to respond with agility and effectiveness. However, local variations did show promise in managing the crisis at a smaller scale, depending on effective leadership and participation, as well as cumulative investments in municipal capacities. The case of Ecuador highlights the significance of pandemic politics in the international political economy. The global governance of public health has led to significant health inequalities, both locally and globally, due to power disparities in access to healthcare. Dysfunctions in global health governance contribute to this unequal status quo.

In Mexico, the causes of the weak response can be found in the convergence created by the introduction of a failed health reform at virtually the same moment when the pandemic struck, as well as the existence of a federal government incapable and reluctant to develop social and policy learning processes essential to formulate an effective response to any crisis (Dunlop and Radaelli, 2018). Incremental improvements to healthcare provision since the early 2000s were abruptly undermined by the government that took office in late 2018, while despite the official rhetoric, historical deficiencies and inequalities not only were not reduced but were exacerbated. Rather than making progress towards the creation of a unified, effective, and efficient public healthcare system, its previous historical fragmentation was reproduced with the mere substitution of the voluntary health insurance programme for labour market outsiders, with a programme that intended to adopt universal principles by offering access as a citizenship right but that in practice represented a case of welfare retrenchment. The supply of tertiary care for informal sector workers and their families was eliminated, policy rules that established access and care for that population group were cancelled without publishing new rules, and the medicines procurement system for the entire public sector was dismantled without creating a new system that could meet demand.

The centralisation and politicisation of the management of the pandemic in Mexico shielded domestic policy from the influence of global policies emitted by the WHO, PAHO, and other international organisations. The government's inability to incorporate new knowledge that was emerging from international actors and organisations as the pandemic unfolded into its own response had grave consequences for the Mexican people. Populist polarisation can lead governments to act dogmatically, refusing dialogue with any social or political actor not aligned with their own decisions and preferences. International actors are commonly viewed with suspicion, as they tend to be considered representatives of foreign interests. However, when adopting this perspective, governments only end up damaging their populations, denying them the formulation and implementation of policy solutions necessary to address their social problems.

Conclusion

The analysis presented in this chapter shows the blurred lines between government and governance in contemporary policymaking. Current problems that threaten the well-being of societies have causes and consequences that transcend national spheres. The assumption that domestic government actors have the capacity to solve them on their own without collaborations with foreign actors is simply an illusion. The collaboration between national and international state and non-state actors is necessary to formulate and implement the public policies necessary to protect people from the risks posed by global shocks like the COVID-19 pandemic. Transnational governance structures should have the capacity to endow global policy with the potential to influence national policy for the benefit of the people.

The comparative analysis of Ecuador and Mexico reveals the contradictions and limitations of global policies concerning pandemic politics. In the economic realm, foreign actors can impose a policy course on a national government, as observed in Ecuador, where the IMF urged for public spending cuts during economic difficulties. However, in the health and social realms, international organisations can only potentially influence domestic policymaking spaces through deliberation and learning processes. When confronted with a populist government, as in Mexico, the possibility of developing those processes is likely to fail. This demonstrates the procedural and instrumental aspects of pandemic responses, where global policies must generate a better balance and coordination between economic and social policy, as well as a more energetic intervention in the latter. Unless this is done, it is difficult to envision how national healthcare systems could be strengthened to face health crises like the COVID-19 pandemic. It is worth highlighting how governance and governmental actors have often failed to address pandemic politics, with dire human consequences. The comparative case studies of Ecuador and Mexico illustrate how global policies have struggled to develop effective pandemic responses and how domestic political systems can impede international organisations' ability to influence policymaking in the health and social realms.

The chapter has discussed how, even if formal compliance with international regulations was reported prior to the pandemic, the response in both cases was hampered by the symbolic nature of the decisions taken by political actors—who did not seem to abandon their preoccupation with avoiding political losses during the health crises—the failure or absence of adequate disease diplomacy—as in the case of Ecuador, where pressures from the global financial sphere contradicted the ability to meet policy recommendations from the global health sphere—the effects of medical populism—of which the Mexican response can even represent a model case—and the political economy of health systems, with deep inequalities in the supply and access to health services by different socio-economic groups in both countries. Global economic policy seems to have the coercive capacity to shape national policy. Existing governance arrangements give international organisations the power to condition financial support for the adoption of economic reforms that limit the dynamic capabilities of the public sector to manage a crisis. Though reforms are justified to stabilise national finances, there is an apparent absence of coordination between financial and social policy organisations, like the ones governing global healthcare, that, especially in times of crises, yields devastating consequences, as happened in Ecuador during the pandemic. At the same time, the health crisis revealed the ineffectiveness of global policy in steering national decision-making processes, when the adoption of emergency measures devised with the knowledge generated by transnational actors is fundamental to protecting people's well-being. In fact, and as noted by Mazzucato and Kattel (2020), the global rules that govern sectors such as health since the early 2000s have made punitive use of intellectual property that limits the capacity to respond during deep crises. Global crises like the pandemic, as well as others that can be foreseen in the near future, require a much better coordinated and more effective global policy.

Notes

1 The previous version of the IHR dated back to 1969 and was restricted to activities related to the prevention and treatment of only cholera, plague, and yellow fever (Rodier *et al.*, 2007).
2 The use of private services is also incentivised by the deductions from income tax of private health spending, including private insurance and out-of-pocket spending.
3 The central role assumed by the UHPP was enhanced when other offices of the SS were eliminated or fused, part of the austerity plan adopted by the federal government when it took office in late 2018. For example, the previously autonomous regulatory agency for health treatments and medicines was put under the authority of the UPPS. The centralisation of functions created problems for the management of public healthcare provision on several fronts, not only in response to the pandemic (IGHS, 2021).
4 The acquisition of COVID-19 vaccines has been one area in which the leadership was not assigned to the UHPP but the Secretariat for Foreign Relations. It is not clear why that decision was made, but in any case, that could well be the only area where the government's response can be classified as successful since the number of vaccines from different companies has been plentiful (IGHS, 2021).
5 The interventions covered were pregnancies, births, and puerperium; caesarean deliveries; diseases of the appendix; complicated hernias; complicated gastric and duodenal ulcers; endoscopies; and cholecystectomies. In some states, specific agreements were signed for the provision of some private services to COVID-19 patients, like in Mexico City, but they were not extended to the entire country (SS, 2020).
6 Of the total number of people who reported to have had at least one symptom, 58% sought medical care and 43% received it in the private sector (INSP, 2021).

7 González Block et al. (2020) estimate a rate of 1.9 doctors per 1,000 population in Mexico based on national employment surveys, lower than the rate reported by the OECD.

References

Agren, D. (2020) 'Understanding Mexican health worker COVID-19 deaths', *The Lancet*, 396(10254), p. 807.

Altmann, P., King, K., Maldonado, R. and Polo Bonilla, R. (2020) *Covid-19 in Ecuador. Feelings, attitudes, socioeconomic effects*. Quito: Central University of Ecuador.

Bambra, C., Lynch, J. and Smith, K. (2021) *The unequal pandemic. COVID-19 and health inequalities*. Bristol: Bristol University Press.

BBC (2020) 'Coronavirus: Ecuador struggles to bury its victims', [En línea]. Available at: https://www.bbc.com/news/av/ world-latin-america-52234127.

Bernales-Baksai, P. and Velázquez Leyer, R. (2021) 'In search of the "authentic" universalism in Latin American healthcare: a comparison of policy architectures and outputs in Chile and Mexico', *Journal of Comparative Policy Analysis: Research and Practice*, 24(4), pp. 385–405.

Bonilla-Chacín, M. and Aguilera, N. (2013) *The Mexican social protection system in health. Universal health coverage studies series no. 1*. The World Bank.

Büscher, B., Feola, G., Fischer, A., Fletcher, R., Gerber, J.F., Harcourt, W., Koster, M., Schneider, M., Scholtens, J., Spierenburg, M., Walstra, V. and Wiskerke, H. (2021) 'Planning for a world beyond COVID-19: five pillars for post-neoliberal development', *World Development*, 140, 105357.

Carpio, N. (2001) *Alcance y procesos de las reformas de los sistemas de salud en Ecuador*. [Online]. Available at: www.oecd.org/els/health-systems/health-expenditure.htm#:~:text=Preliminary%20estimates%20for%20a%20group,on%20health%20accelerated%20to%204.9%25.&text=Despite%20the%20post%2Dcrisis%20slowdown,of%20health%20systems%20remain%20large (Accessed 3 January 2024).

CDES (2020) 'La vida antes que la deuda: decisiones urgentes para enfrentar el Covid 19'. Available at: http://cdes.org.ec/ web/la-vida-antes-que-la-deuda-decisiones-urgentes-para-enfrentar-el-covid-19/.

COE (2020) 'Protocolo de Comunicación y atención de casos de violencia de género e intrafamiliar en la emergencia por coronavirus (COVID-19)'. Available at: https://www.gestionderiesgos.gob.ec/wp-content/uploads/2020/07/05.PRT04_Protcontra Violencia-signed.pdf.

CONADIS (2020) 'CONADIS lanza guía para la atención de las personas con discapacidad debido a la emergencia sanitaria'. Available at: https://www.consejodiscapacidades. gob.ec/conadis-lanza-guia-para-la-atencion-de-laspersonas-con-discapacidad-debido-a-la-emergencia-sanitaria/.

Consejo Nacional para la Igualdad de Pueblos y Nacionalidades (2020) 'Protocolo con pertinencia intercultural para la prevención y atención de la covid-19 en pueblos y nacionalidades indígenas, afroecuatorianos y montubios del Ecuador'. Available at: http://www.pueblosynacionalidades.gob.ec/wp-content/uploads/2020/08/ PROTOCOLOPUEBLOS_Y_NACIONALIDADES_APROBADO_COE.pdf.

Díaz Pabón, F.A. and Palacio Ludeña, M.G. (2021) 'Inequality and the socioeconomic dimensions of mobility in protests: the cases of Quito and Santiago', *Global Policy*, 12, pp. 78–90.

Dunlop, C.A. and Radaelli, C.M. (2018) 'The lessons of policy learning: types, triggers, hindrances and pathologies', *Policy & Politics*, 46(2), pp. 255–72.

El Comercio (2020a) 'COE nacional pidió coordinar normas entre municipalidades luego del estado de excepción'. Available at: https://www.elcomercio.com/actualidad/coe-normas-municipios-excepcion.html.

El Comercio (2020b) 'Manifestantes recorren este 22 de octubre del 2020 la avenida 9 de Octubre de Guayaquil'. Available at: https://www.elcomercio.com/actualidad/manifestantes-guayaquil-protesta-politicas-economicas.html.

El Comercio (2020c) 'Solo un Municipio emitió sanción por aglomeración'. Available at: https://www.elcomercio.com/ actualidad/municipios-sanciones-aglomeraciones-elecciones-protocolo.html.

Espinosa, V. *et al.* (2017) 'La reforma en salud del Ecuador', *Revista Panamericana de Salud Pública*, 41.

Financial Times (2020a) 'Coronavirus tracked: the latest figures as countries fight Covid-19 resurgence'. Available at: https://www.ft.com/content/a2901ce8-5eb7-4633-b89c-cbdf5b386938.

Financial Times (2020b) 'Ecuador clinches $17.4bn debt deal with bondholders'. Available at: https://www.ft.com/content/567d51c2-4410-4fdd-a59b-7227077cb922.

Financial Times (2020c) 'Ecuador reaches deal to postpone debt repayments until August'. Available at: https://www.ft.com/ content/e1622284-102c-48f0-b45d-dadb 81579d9d.

Financial Times (2020d) '"This is a real world war": Ecuador's president on the virus'. Available at: https://www.ft.com/ content/98faa3c9-d4ab-4974-95fd-eeca519cd8c9.

GHS INDEX (2021) *Global health security index*. Johns Hopkins Center for Health Security, Nuclear Threat Initiative (NTI). [Online]. Available at: www.ghsindex.org/ (Accessed 3 January 2024).

Goldman, M. (2009) *La descentralización del sistema de salud del Ecuador: un estudio comparativo de "Espacio de Decisión" y capacidad entre los sistemas municipales de salud de Quito, Guayaquil y Cuenca*. Quito: FLACSO-Ecuador.

González Block, M. *et al.* (2018) *El subsistema privado de atención de la salud en México. Diagnóstico y Retos*. Naucalpan de Juárez: Universidad Anáhuac.

González Block, M. *et al.* (2020) *Mexico health system review. North American observatory on health systems and policies (NAO)*. Copenhagen: World Health Organization.

IGHS (2021) *La respuesta de México al COVID-19: Estudio de caso*. San Francisco: Institute for Global Health Sciences—University of California.

INEC (2019) *Registro Estadístico de Recursos y Actividades de Salud*. Instituto Nacional de Estadística y Censos. Available at: www.ecuadorencifras.gob.ec/actividades-y-recursos-de-salud/ (Accessed 10 January 2024).

INEGI (2017) *Encuesta Nacional de Empleo y Seguridad Social (ENESS) 2017*. Instituto Nacional de Geografía y Estadística. [Online]. Available at: www.inegi.org.mx/programas/eness/2017/ (Accessed 10 January 2024).

INSABI (2020, 12 December) *Programa Institucional 2020–2024 del Instituto Nacional de Salud para el Bienestar*. Diario Oficial de la Federación.

INSP (2021) *Encuesta Nacional de Salud y Nutrición 2020 sobre COVID-19. Resultados Nacionales*. Instituto Nacional de Salud Pública.

Jiménez-Barbosa, W.G. *et al.* (2017) 'Transformaciones del sistema de salud ecuatoriano', *Universidad y Salud*, 19(1), pp. 126–139.

King, K., Altmann, P. and Polo Bonilla, R. (2020) 'LSE blogs: Ecuador's mishandled COVID-19 health crisis has also had serious economic, educational, and emotional impacts'. Available at: https://blogs.lse.ac.uk/latamcaribbean/2020/11/18/ecuadors-mishandled-covid-19-health-crisis-has-also-had-serious-economic-educational-and-emotional-impacts/.

Lucio, R., López, R., Leines, N. and Terán, J.A. (2019) 'El financiamiento de la salud en Ecuador', *Revista PUCE*, 108. https://doi.org/10.26807/revpuce.v0i108.215.

Lucio, R., Villacrés, H. and Henríquez, R. (2011) 'Sistema de salud de Ecuador', *Salud Pública de México (Instituto Nacional de Salud Pública)*, 53(2), pp. S177–S187.

Martínez Franzoni, J. and Sánchez Ancochea, D. (2016) *The quest for universal social policy in the South. Actors, ideas and architectures.* Cambridge: Cambridge University Press.

Mazzucato, M. and Kattel, R. (2020) 'COVID-19 and public-sector capacity', *Oxford Review of Economic Policy*, 36(1), pp. 256–269.

Mesa-Lago, C. (2005) *Las reformas de salud en América Latina y el Caribe: su impacto en los principios de la seguridad social. Documentos de proyectos.* Comisión Económica para América Latina y el Caribe (CEPAL).

Naciones Unidas (2020) *Plan de Respuesta Humanitaria Covid-19 Ecuador*, Naciones Unidas—Equipo Humanitario de País. Available at: https://reliefweb.int/report/ecuador/plan-de-respuesta-humanitaria-covid-19-ecuadorequipo-humanitario-de-pa-s-abril-2020 (Accessed 15 April 2021).

Naranjo, S. (2020) 'Google data'. Available at: https://datastudio.google.com/reporti ng/937828fd-93f2-4ff1-a260- e6cdb458d1d2/page/TBdZB.

New York Times (2020). 'Ecuador's death toll during outbreak is among the worst in the world', Available at: https://www. nytimes.com/2020/04/23/world/americas/ecuador-deaths-coronavirus.html.

Nigenda, G. *et al.* (2015) 'Evaluating the implementation of Mexico's health reform: the case of Seguro popular', *Health Systems & Reform*, 1(3), pp. 217–228.

Observatorio Social (2020, 8 September). *El Acceso geográfico desigual a la salud en Ecuador.* COVID-19 Ecuador. [Online]. Available at: www.covid19ecuador.org/post/salud-publica-pandemia-2 (Accessed 10 January 2024).

OEA (2016) *Informe Nacional sobre la implementación del Protocolo de San Salvador.* Washington, DC: Misión Permanente del Ecuador ante la Organización de los Estados Americanos.

OECD (2016) *OECD reviews of health systems: Mexico.* Paris: OECD Publishing.

OECD (2021) *Health at a glance 2021: OECD indicators. Highlights for Mexico.* Organisation for Economic Co-Operation and Development.

OECD (2022) *OECD data. Health.* [Online]. Available at: https://data.oecd.org/health.htm (Accessed 11 January 2024).

OIT (2021) *El sistema de salud ecuatoriano y la COVID-19.* Nota Informativa OIT Países Andinos.

OPS/OMS. (2007) *La equidad en la mira: la salud pública en Ecuador durante las últimas décadas.* Quito: OPS/MSP/CONASA.

Palacio Ludeña, M.G. (2023) 'The health care system in Ecuador', *Social Policy Country Briefs.* Bremen: SFB Globale Entwicklungsdynamiken von Sozialpolitik.

Plan-V (2020) '*Pandemia: las cifras „variables" que confunden a los alcaldes*'. Available at: https://www.planv.com.ec/ historias/sociedad/pandemia-cifras-variables-que-confunden-alcaldes.

Progressive International (2020) 'IMF austerity is strangling Ecuador – again'. Available at: https://progressive.international/ wire/2020-12-14-the-imfs-austerity-is-strangling-ecuador--again/en.

Puertas Donoso, B., Herrera Herrera, M. and Aguinaga, G. (2004) 'La Promoción de Salud en el Ecuador', in *La Promoción de Salud en América Latina: modelos, estructuras y visión crítica.* San Juan: Centre for Disease Control.

Reich, M. (2020) 'Restructuring health reform, Mexican style', *Health Systems & Reform*, 6(1).

Rodier, G. *et al.* (2007) 'Global public health security', *Emerging Infectious Diseases*, 13(10), pp. 1447–1452.

SS (2020) 'Todos juntos contra el COVID'. [Online]. Available at: https://coronavirus. gob.mx/todos-juntos/ (Accessed 12 January 2024).

Thomas, S. *et al.* (2020) *Strengthening health systems resilience: key concepts and strategies, policy brief 36, European observatory on health systems and policies.* World Health Organization.

Ulloa, E. *et al.* (2020) 'Descifrar el Modelo Centinela', *Nexos—Taller de datos.* [Online]. Available at: https://datos.nexos.com.mx/descifrando-el-modelo-centinel a/ (Accessed 16 July 2023).

WHO (2011) *Strengthening national health emergency and disaster management capacities and resilience of health systems.* Agenda item 4.5 22, Sixty-fourth World Health Assembly 128th Session, World Health Organization EB128/SR/10.

WHO (2021) *Health topics—international health regulations.* World Health Organization. [Online]. Available at: www.who.int/health-topics/international-health-regulations#tab=tab_1 (Accessed 12 January 2024).

WHO (2022) *WHO coronavirus (COVID-19) dashboard.* World Health Organization. [Online]. Available at: https://covid19.who.int/ (Accessed 12 January 2024).

World Health Organization (2021) 'Global health expenditure database'. *NHA Indicators.* Available at: https://apps.who.int/nha/database/ViewData/Indicators/en (Accessed 15 April 2021).

7 Limitations of Collaborative Governance Within Mexico's Highly Disbalanced Federalist System

Heidi Jane M. Smith

Introduction

The global spread of SARS-CoV-2, known as COVID-19, revealed the vulnerabilities of healthcare systems worldwide. In Mexico, a federalist country, the response to the pandemic also exposed significant institutional weaknesses, marked by high death and case rates.[1] President López Obrador played a significant role in downplaying the pandemic early on, consistently expressing scepticism about its existence. He often criticised the use of masks and deferred policy responses, contributing to a delayed reaction to the unfolding crisis.[2] His reluctance led to opposition leaders proposing policy solutions already long applied in the United States, Italy, China, and the United Kingdom.

The Federalist Alliance, comprised of ten governors from diverse political backgrounds, played a pivotal role in the pandemic politics that occurred. Opposition governors from the National Action Party (PAN), the Institutional Revolutionary Party (PRI), the Citizen Movement (MC), and the Party of the Democratic Revolution (PRD) united in their criticism of the federal government's public management response, and particularly the president's inaction before the pandemic. Their coordinated efforts, particularly by states like Jalisco, Aguascalientes, Queretaro, and San Luis Potosí, led to the formation of the Alianza Centro-Bajío-Occidente, a central region of the country. This regional alliance aimed to address the pandemic collectively, implementing measures such as reinforcing testing stations and supporting key industries to sustain the economy. In September 2020, these state governors decided to withdraw from the National Conference of Governors, citing its ineffectiveness and failure to defend state sovereignty. Simultaneously, opposition governors, part of the Alianza Centro-Bajío-Occidente and the Alianza Federalista, argued for a "new Federalism" system grounded in a revised fiscal pact. Their contention was rooted in the perceived lack of a rational response to the pandemic and a viable plan for economic reactivation.

The ensuing power struggle influenced the July 2021 midterm elections, where 500 seats in the Chamber of Deputies and 15 governorships were contested. Despite opposition parties holding 14 governorships, President López

DOI: 10.4324/9781003494959-7

Obrador's MORENA (National Regeneration Movement) party emerged victorious, shifting the balance of power in their favour. Also, MORENA maintained its majority in the Chamber of Deputies but fell short of the qualified majority needed to unilaterally amend the constitution. The coalition led by MORENA, including the Workers' Party (PT) and the Green Party (PVEM), secured the most seats, reflecting a diverse political landscape without a single dominant party. Ultimately, the 2021 midterm elections did not bring a significant change to the power of the president or his mandate, with the ruling party retaining control over the legislative branch and a majority of the governorships, eventually strengthening his control over the central government.

So why did the Federalist Alliance revolt not alter electoral politics more substantially? This chapter delves into the dynamics of the weak federal response, shedding light on the emergence of pandemic politics as governors challenged the status quo during a critical period and lost. To do this, it critically analyses the impact of the COVID-19 pandemic policies implemented in Mexico by reviewing the government's attempt at a more collaborative governance approach and drawing attention to the complexities of federalism, with its high levels of inequality within and between states and overall low levels of state capacity.

Presidentialism and the Opening of Democracy With Decentralisation

The Federal Republic of Mexico issued its first constitution in 1824. Since then, the 32 states that make up the Mexican territory are individual sovereigns with varying abilities to implement public policies. Article 115 in the 1917 constitution outlines the responsibilities of local governments to provide public services like water supply, lighting, public safety, and local transportation, while allowing them autonomy to regulate urban development, land use planning, and encourage local tax collection. In practice, the country has taken almost 200 years to consolidate power and centralise control, thanks to the one-party hegemonic power of the Institutional Revolutionary Party (PRI), which held the presidency for more than 80 years.

In Mexico, *presidentialism*, defined by Weldon (1997), allows the head of state to exercise an extraordinary range of powers. For example, in the past, presidents could reform the constitution by proposing amendments with little influence from Congress. They could propose the legislation necessary to be successful throughout their six-year term, and they could even appoint their own successor to the presidency. Likewise, the president could nominate most of the candidates for Congress from his party, some governors, mayors, and members of Congress, including his cabinet, as well as obedient representatives of the judiciary. However, due to several constitutional reforms, the control of the president is now much less than before the beginning of the new century.

In general, these changes signified Mexico's dedication to adapting its constitution to contemporary public policy challenges, spanning from representation to education, transparency, and healthcare. For example, political reforms in the electoral process aimed to enhance democracy, transparency, and citizen participation. Amendments focusing on human and indigenous rights address historical injustices and promote cultural diversity. The 2013 education reform introduced standardised evaluations and merit-based promotions. Criminal justice reforms enhanced transparency and human rights protection. In 2013, energy reforms opened up the sector to foreign investment. Healthcare and fiscal federalism reforms in 2019 aimed to establish universal healthcare and redistribute resources equitably. With the transition to democracy, Mexico entered a new public policy dynamic, which was represented by the alternation between political parties. Lehoucq *et al.* (2005) described how changes in the public policy process were very slow after democratisation but quickly increased after these constitutional reforms.

Like many Latin American countries, Mexico initiated a democratisation process in the 1980s in response to the authoritarian governments in the 1970s and 1980s. This transition involved local elections and the delegation of responsibilities to local governments, emphasising public services, health, and education programmes (Rosenbaum and Rodriguez Acosta, 2008). This decentralisation aimed at enhancing efficiency and responsiveness to local needs, granting state and municipal governments increased budget authority and autonomy (Smith and Revell, 2016). The decentralisation process countered authoritarianism by fostering improved citizen-government relationships, accountability measures, and pluralistic decision-making.

In the specific case of Mexico, this democratic transition began in 1989 with the triumph of the National Action Party (PAN) in the elections for Governor of Baja California, putting an end to the single-party government of the PRI. The alternation caused reforms to promote fiscal decentralisation, which paradoxically caused a greater dependence of the states on the federal government in fiscal matters but with greater administrative and political autonomy (Smith, 2018). The regulatory framework for the distribution of federal resources, as well as a dynamic of formal cooperation between subnational governments and the federal government, is established in the Fiscal Coordination Law (LCF), issued in 1978. This law describes how federal resources are distributed among the states (known in Mexico as federal entities).

The spending decentralisation reforms in 1993 led to the creation of budget item 28 (also known as *participaciones*) as a mandatory transfer to the states, and budget item 33 (known as *aportaciones*), conditional transfers to the states from the federal government, and an introduction of the value-added tax for federal collection (Rodríguez, 1998). Finally, and most importantly, the reforms of Article 115 gave municipalities the responsibility to provide public services with their own resources and the ability to generate debt. Intergovernmental fiscal federalism in Mexico still faces challenges stemming from an unequal vertical fiscal structure and subnational dependency on federal transfers (Hernández-Trillo, 2018).

Fiscal reforms initiated in the early 2000s sought to address these issues with lasting consequences. Noteworthy reforms include the 2003 fiscal reform, which aimed to empower local governments using over 300 fiscal arrangements negotiated directly with the Ministry of Finance (Pérez Benítez and Villarreal Páez, 2018). The 2007 Fiscal Coordination Law reform refocused the federal share of conditional and unconditional arrangements, encouraging incentives and more fiscal autonomy to states with larger tax bases like Nuevo Leon, Guanajuato, and Guadalajara (Smith, 2018). The National Law of Fiscal Discipline, enforced in 2016 at the state level and 2018 at the municipal level, aimed to control subnational debt issuances (Jimenez Quiroga and Smith, 2019). Despite encouraging signs of growth, concerns persist about the increasing dependence on conditional and unconditional transfers without substantial effects on economic growth (Mendoza-Velázquez, 2018).

Healthcare Decentralisation in Mexico

In the 1980s, Mexico also witnessed a significant transformation in its health policy, characterised by decentralisation reforms and the establishment of the Ministry of Health (Secretaría de Salud) in 1983. A key reform during this period was the decentralisation of health services, involving the transfer of responsibility from the federal government to state and local governments. This shift aimed to enhance the responsiveness of healthcare delivery to local needs, with the creation of health jurisdictions (*jurisdicciones sanitarias*) granting local authorities increased control over health planning and resource allocation. These reforms laid the foundation for a more responsive and inclusive healthcare system in Mexico, encompassing centralised health policymaking with the introduction of social protection mechanisms. In general, decentralisation of services put an emphasis on primary healthcare and encouraged the implementation of robust information systems. Together, these initiatives shaped a transformative vision for the nation's health sector, addressing local needs while fostering efficiency and inclusivity.

In that same era, the groundwork for the System of Social Protection in Health (Sistema de Protección Social en Salud), commonly known as Seguro Popular, was established and later implemented in the early 2000s. In 2003, the significant "Seguro Popular" programme was launched, specifically addressing individuals without formal employment or social security. This initiative aimed at expanding healthcare coverage for underserved populations, aligning with the overarching goal of achieving universal healthcare (Moreno Jaimes, Rojas-Alvarez and Angel, 2023). Recent comprehensive healthcare reforms have further transformed Seguro Popular into "Salud para el Bienestar," placing emphasis on a holistic well-being approach and improving healthcare access, particularly for vulnerable populations.

Today, Mexico's health system is overseen by three key agencies. The Ministry of Health (Secretaría de Salud—SSA), established in 1983, is the principal federal entity responsible for developing and implementing national health policies, emphasising disease prevention and health promotion. The Mexican Social Security Institute (Instituto Mexicano del Seguro Social—IMSS) provides healthcare services to formal sector employees and their dependents, offering a range of benefits from medical care to pensions. Another important institution is the Institute of Security and Social Services for State Workers (Instituto de Seguridad y Servicios Sociales de los Trabajadores del Estado—ISSSTE), catering to the health and social needs of government employees (Moreno Jaimes, Rojas-Alvarez and Angel, 2023). Together, these agencies contribute to Mexico's healthcare landscape, each playing a distinct role in ensuring widespread health coverage for the population. Presidential coordination mechanisms, including the National Health Council (CNS) and intersectoral health committees, play pivotal roles in policy formulation and collaboration.

Curiously, during the pandemic, President López Obrador reformed the CNS, transforming it into two additional councils. The Consejo de Salubridad General (CSG) oversees the health regulations and intergovernmental relations between states and the federal government, while the Consejo Nacional de Salud para el Bienestar was set to focus on national health and well-being more globally (Knaul et al., 2023). However, challenges arose with the new governance structure, as federal resources were not proportionally increased, requiring the government to navigate the health crisis with limited financial support (Frenk and Gómez Dantés, 2020; Periódico el Heraldo, 2021).[3]

Asymmetric Decentralisation and the Devolution of Decision-Making at the Local Level

Fiscal federalism, distinct from fiscal decentralisation, involves the national government sharing revenues with lower levels, aiming for effective public policies (Tanzi, 2000). The first wave of reforms in the 1980s focused on decentralising electoral responsibility, taxing authority, and introducing results-based budgeting (Wiesner, 2003). However, flawed targeted fiscal transfers and conditional welfare policies emerged. The second-generation reforms, starting in the late 1990s, integrated microeconomics into decentralisation, emphasising market-based incentives (Wiesner, 2003). Mexico's decentralisation aimed at improving service delivery but paradoxically increased fiscal dependence on the federal government (Rosenbaum and Rodriguez Acosta, 2008). A challenge is the lack of local government incentives to collect taxes, relying on central transfers. Known by academics as the soft bailout problem, high vertical imbalances and moral hazards still persist in Mexico (Diaz-Cayeros, 2006; Hernández-Trillo, 2018) and were exacerbated by the COVID-19 pandemic. Admittedly, acknowledging these heterogeneous effects, known as asymmetric decentralisation, may enhance fiscal and administrative capacity in the long term (Tan and Avshalom-Uster, 2021).

In a federalist state like Mexico, fiscal agreements between the national and subnational governments are crucial. This complex web of governance helps explain how Mexico is managed. The nature of fiscal federalism involves defining competencies between different levels of the Federation for tax collection and public spending (Pliego Moreno, 2012). The system theoretically allows for more efficient resource allocation at the local level, considering specific needs. Local governments, with closer contact and better data, can offer goods and services at lower costs, strengthening fiscal responsibility within the Federation (Gandarilla, 2012). Conversely, centralising these functions may overlook specific population needs, resulting in a uniform provision of goods without considering local characteristics.

A federalist state has a legal system that combines subnational units of government to report back on their spending. Many of these reporting systems of government have legal agreements. The first article of the Mexican Fiscal Coordination Law establishes that the Mexican Federation will enter into an agreement with each of its Federative Entities (States) to adhere to the National Fiscal Coordination System through the Ministry of Finance (Secretaría de Hacienda y Crédito Público). The Mexican Fiscal System establishes what resources are paid and received through public funds between the states and the federal government. As can be seen, "the nature of fiscal federalism implies a definition of competencies between the different levels of the Federation to carry out tax collection and public spending" (Pliego Moreno, 2012). The problem is that several states do not have sufficient competencies or resources to add additional funds for policymaking.

In theory, this system fosters increased citizen welfare as the Federation collects and distributes the public resources, which each state allocates more efficiently, as long as at the local level it has more contact with people and data to better understand their needs. Doing this can be considered to be cheaper, as local governments offer goods and services to the population at the lowest cost. While performing this task, the federal government will expect local governments to strengthen their fiscal responsibility as members of a Federation (Gandarilla, 2012). On the other hand, if the central government had those functions, specific needs would be unknown, so it would probably provide the same amount and type of goods to the entire population without considering their particular needs and peculiar characteristics.

In practice, Mexico is a highly unequal society, and its Federation reflects that; it is less like the United States federation, which it is said to reflect. The current type of federalism in Mexico has *become increasingly unbalanced*, as many states, particularly in the South and Southeast, are highly dependent on federal resources. Indeed, Gandarilla (2012) suggested that Mexican federalism continues to be highly centralised in terms of income and increasingly decentralised spending. This imbalance may be corrected through mechanisms of joint responsibility between the Federation and states in issues related to public finances and the establishment of guidelines and regulations in the case of debt contracting, for example. This *unbalanced system of fiscal federalism* has had an effect on states' and municipal governments' ability to implement quality public policies. The consequences of this imbalance were evident during the COVID-19 pandemic, as the largest number of patients and deaths were concentrated in highly populated states in the north and centre of the country, like Mexico City, Chihuahua, Baja California, and Sonora, which present much more cases than in the rest of the country. Because of this demand for services from these states with the most population, less was available for other states. Indeed, if these states were omitted from an analysis, COVID-19 cases seem to be distributed in a more balanced way.

Collaborative Governance and Hypothesis Tests

Therefore, decentralisation, aiming to enhance citizen well-being, relies on the central government's resource collection and redistribution to address local needs. Failure in this process, termed "government failure" by Oates (1972), as observed in the COVID-19 pandemic, exposes flaws in public goods allocation. The state's limited influence on economic policy, constrained by central bank independence and capital market investments, for example (Bodea and Hicks, 2015; Mosley, 2000), necessitates organised public policy and finances. Sour (2008) emphasises an economic approach to policy design and evaluation. In her research, Mosley (2000) explores the impact of capital market openness on government policies, noting that while international financial markets strongly influence governments, their impact is narrow. Central to this debate is the government's role in function execution and resource collection, necessitating redistribution to local governments.

The discussion emphasises that effective governance requires collaboration and coordination between different levels of government. Collaborative governance models, as studied by Cyr *et al.* (2021), become crucial in this context. The study reveals that while Mexico ranked high in institutional collaboration (74%), indicating effective collaboration within institutions, it ranked mid-level in terms of inter-governmental collaboration (54%). This underscores a challenge in coordinating efforts between various levels of government, reflecting potential issues in decentralised systems. Pointing towards the importance of collaborative governance for a more cohesive and effective response may seem idealistic, especially during crises like the pandemic.

For example, the study by Rogers et al. (2021) on COVID-19 highlighted disparities within Mexico, emphasising economic and physical inequalities among states and cities within the federal system. Using mobility data from five Mexican cities, it explored the link between local income, education, and behaviours associated with COVID-19 risk post-national lockdowns. Despite higher COVID-19 risks for low-income individuals, evidence on whether people in low-income urban areas engage in riskier behaviour was mixed. In a broader Latin American context, Ramírez de la Cruz *et al.* (2020) assessed transaction costs for governmental responses to COVID-19. By analysing actions in Argentina, Brazil, Chile, Colombia, and Mexico, the authors found limited professionalisation, especially in less developed, corrupt cities, and constrained financial resources for implementing policies. The study also highlighted the extraordinary political risk aversion in urban regions, making it challenging to implement recommendations and causing tension across government levels.

Hegele and Schnabel (2021) proposed a federalism evaluation framework using a 2x2 quadrant analysis, examining centralised or decentralised decision-making in crisis management. Analysing Austria, Germany, and Switzerland, they observed variations in coordination levels and decision-making authority. Their study suggested that federal governments internalised negative externalities like competition and citizen complaints in their pandemic responses. The authors' analytical framework provides insights into the diverse approaches taken by governments in responding to the COVID-19 crisis, contributing to a deeper understanding of crisis management within the context of federalism. Their model is outlined in Table 7.1.

The table distinguishes between unilateral decision-making, where the federal government decides without coordinating with states, and coordinated decision-making, where the federal government involves states in either a top-down or bottom-up coordination approach. Similarly, the table outlines scenarios where states make decisions independently or coordinate horizontally with other states or vertically with the federal government. Adapted from Hegele and Schnabel (2021), the model suggests a collaborative governance structure that expands decision-making capacities, allowing for a spectrum from bottom-up to top-down decision-making and contrasting unilateral decisions with coordinated approaches.[4]

This research builds on the framework outlined in Table 7.1, proposing the hypothesis that the effectiveness of public policies at the state level

Table 7.1 Federalism and COVID-19 crisis management analysis

Centralised decision-making		
Unilateral decision-making	Federal government decides without coordinating with states.	Federal government coordinates with states when deciding (top down).	**Coordinating decision-making**
	States decide without coordinating with other states or federal government.	States coordinate with other states (horizontal coordination) or federal government when deciding (bottom-up coordination).	
Decentralised decision-making		

Source: Adapted from Hegele and Schnabel (2021)

during the COVID-19 crisis is significantly influenced by coordination levels in decision-making authority. States with centralised decision-making structures (high coordination level) may demonstrate more uniform policy implementation, potentially leading to better crisis management outcomes. In contrast, states with decentralised decision-making structures (low coordination level) may exhibit diverse policy responses, resulting in disparities in the impact of COVID-19 across regions. The collaborative governance structure identified in Table 7.1, allowing for a spectrum from bottom-up to top-down decision-making, is anticipated to play a pivotal role in shaping state-level policies and determining their effectiveness in addressing the challenges posed by the pandemic. This is simplified in Table 7.2.

The main purpose of this research is to evaluate the relationship between the effectiveness of public policies at the state level during the COVID-19 crisis and coordination levels in decision-making authority. If the states are effective at mitigating the effects of the pandemic, then they were successful at coordinating their decision-making authority among other states and between levels of the federal government. The dependent variable, effectiveness of public policies, is envisioned as a multifaceted measure, encompassing indicators such as the rate of COVID-19 infections, mortality rates, vaccination rates, and economic indicators. Operationalising this variable involves quantifying outcomes such as the percentage reduction in COVID-19 mortality rates, the successful implementation of public health measures, or economic recovery rates.

The independent variable, coordination levels in decision-making authority, serves as a crucial factor influencing the effectiveness of state-level policies. To measure this variable, an assessment of the degree of coordination in decision-making is conducted, ranging from centralised to decentralised structures. For example, operationalisation could entail the creation of a scale or index, where a centralised structure might be scored as 1, a balanced coordination structure as 2, and a decentralised structure as 3. Here, we are providing examples and empirical data from the national statistical agency INEGI based on what happened during the pandemic and their policy outcomes in Mexico.

This comprehensive approach aims to provide a nuanced understanding of the interplay between decision-making coordination, state-level factors, and the effectiveness of public policies in managing the challenges posed by the COVID-19 pandemic.

Table 7.2 How to establish coordination levels versus decision-making authority

Coordination level	Decision-making authority
High	Centralised
Low	Decentralised

Source: Own elaboration

Data Presentation and Analysis

Cited in Chapter 1 of this volume, the Cyr *et al.* (2021) study utilised newspaper clippings to evaluate collaborative governance, emphasising inter-governmental and institutional collaboration in policy planning and implementation. Their research did not delve into the bureaucracies involved or consider both the highly technical and political aspects of public policy-making. Case studies of Argentina, Brazil, and Uruguay were conducted to complement the newspaper analysis. Here, we go beyond the news clippings and evaluate the actual results of the public policy response in Mexico using census data. First, to carry out the national analysis, a sample of the 32 Federative Entities of Mexico was considered, using as dependent variables the infections and deaths of COVID-19 for each of the states. Data presented in Figures 7.1 and 7.2 come from September 2020 (approximately six months after the initial beginning of the pandemic) published in Our World in Data for that day.

The highly populated states with the highest number of cases and deaths were Mexico City and the State of Mexico, whereas other low-density states had varying levels of impact in terms of absolute numbers of cases and death rates. In September 2020, the highest death rates compared to population were Morelos, Sinaloa, and Baja California. On the other hand, the states

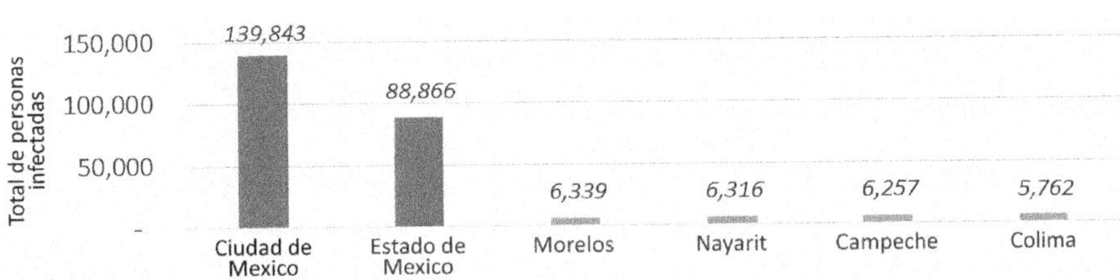

Figure 7.1 Total COVID-19 cases in Mexico in September 2020

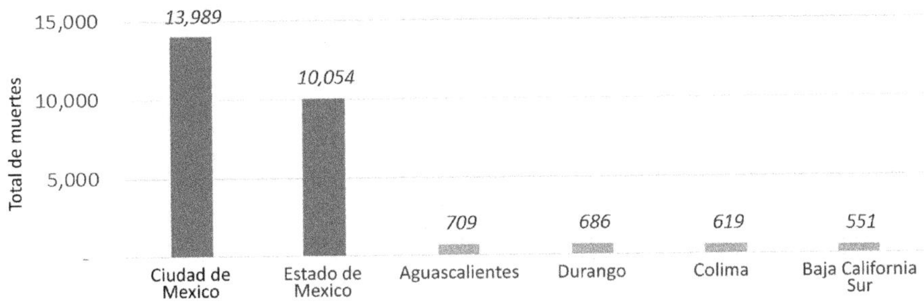

Figure 7.2 Total COVID-19 deaths in Mexico in September 2020

Table 7.3 States with the highest and lowest cases as of September 2020

	State	Cases	Deaths	Relation deaths/cases
Highest rates	Morelos	6,339	1,125	18%
	Sinaloa	19,996	3,398	17%
	Baja California	22,304	3,643	16%
Lowest rates	Coahuila	28,751	2,022	7%
	Durango	10,155	686	7%
	Baja California Sur	11,063	551	5%
	Total México	817,503	83,781	11%

Source: Own elaboration with data from the Ministry of Health COVID-19 database

that had the lowest population rate were Coahuila, Durango, and Baja California Sur, respectively (see Table 7.3).

Yet, measures implemented by states in response to the pandemic varied, with some adopting a diverse array of policies, including support for scholarships, unemployment insurance, aid for COVID-19 patients, labour reintegration, assistance for indigenous people and the elderly, and food support. In contrast, other states focused primarily on food aid and support for vulnerable populations. State-level actions were crucial in addressing the emergency and kickstarting economic recovery. Each of the 32 states in the country designed economic measures tailored to navigate the challenges posed by the pandemic, emphasising the importance of understanding the state-level situation for informed decision-making, but many were insufficient to radically change the economy. Unfortunately, there are few signs of successful collaborative mechanisms.

For example, northern states generally implemented more measures than their southern counterparts, attributed to differences in economic composition and capacity. The social and political conflict during the pandemic extended beyond health concerns to debates about mask wearing. The efficiency of state-level responses, the effectiveness of social programmes, and economic decisions made by state governments had far-reaching consequences, emphasising the importance of analysing the impact of priority social programmes on poverty reduction in both the short and long terms at the state and national levels.

This unbalanced federalism is notable in the analysis of implementing social policies by state-level governments at the same time. In line with previous research on social policy (Medrano, 2016; Medrano and Smith, 2017), much of social policy starts in Mexico City and ends up replicated across other states. In this regard, a clear example to illustrate the federalism imbalance mentioned earlier is Mexico City, a state where power is highly centralised and which shares the same political party as the federal government, MORENA. As seen in Table 7.4, many different public policies were developed early on to face the COVID-19 pandemic in Mexico City, which were replicated later by other states. At the same time, Mexico City had high increases in cases and deaths from COVID-19, so it had to take more drastic measures to fight the pandemic.

These fragmented responses at the subnational level highlight the necessity for a unified approach by the central government. The actions of the Federalist Alliance underscored a collective action problem, reflecting the challenges of coordinating pandemic responses across diverse political landscapes when local control was insufficient. Examining the federalist system, the study emphasised the theoretical benefits of decentralisation, suggesting that local governments, with closer proximity to citizens, can better address their needs. However, practical implementation during the pandemic in Mexico revealed significant imbalances, with income highly centralised and vaccine implementation decentralised in mostly wealthy areas first. This imbalance is evident in the disproportionate concentration of COVID-19 cases and deaths in specific regions.

To combat these high rates of death and cases, the Mexican federal government developed the Federal Vaccination Program against COVID-19, with the aim of inoculating as much of the population as possible. The first injections began at the end of December 2020, starting with the medical sector that worked directly with COVID-19 patients. Subsequently, the programme was implemented by age groups, starting with the elderly. By June 2021, 19% of the population had at least one dose against COVID-19, and 11% were fully vaccinated (see Figure 7.3).

The case study of vaccine distribution in Mexico City highlights shortcomings in the existing federalist system and underscores the necessity for a new system that ensures more equitable policy implementation. Mayor and Head of Government, Claudia Sheinbaum, often noted for exceeding the president's mandate, took initiative and utilised her authority to maximise the well-being of Mexico City's citizens. Specifically, she took charge of vaccine distribution, demonstrating a proactive approach at the local level to address the pressing issue of equitable vaccine access. Yet notable in this initiative was an unequal response by some local governments (*delegations*) to implement the policy.

The vaccination plan began with the adult population (60 years and over). As can be seen in Table 7.5, even at the local level, imbalances were seen when implementing the strategy to address the COVID-19 pandemic. There are some municipalities that have fewer vaccines available than the adult population (60 years and older) that lives there. For example, as of April 12, 2021, Álvaro Obregón had 95,910 vaccines available, while its population (60 years and older) was 128,076. On the other hand, Miguel Hidalgo had 101,950 vaccines available, while its population (60 years and over) was 76,038. The capacity to implement the vaccine exceeded the local authorities' administrative abilities to manage the population, resulting in

Table 7.4 Implementation of public policies in the states with the most (and least) deaths from COVID-19 (data from September 2020)

Type of public policy	States with the most cases of COVID-19		States with the least cases of COVID-19			
	Ciudad de México	Estado de México	Aguascalientes	Durango	Colima	Baja California Sur
Scholarships for students	x					
Unemployment insurance	x					
Support for those infected with COVID-19	x					
Support for employment	x					
Support for indigenous peoples	x					
Supports for older adults	x	x	x	x	x	x
Pantry delivery	x				x	x
Nutritional support	x	x	x	x	x	
Support for vulnerable people		x	x		x	x
Supports for public transport drivers			x			

Source: Own elaboration with information from CIDE

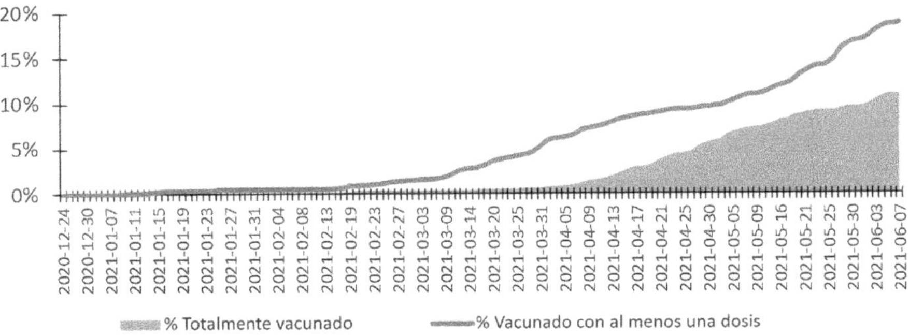

Figure 7.3 Mexicans vaccinated with COVID-19 (as of June 2021)

wealthier populations being attended to first and thereafter less affluent locations.

Another issue was the percentage of coverage by the Mayor's Office (first dose) in Mexico City. While in the wealthier district of Cuajimalpa, 109% were injected, a more populated and less advantaged district, Iztapalapa, had a lower percentage of coverage of only 74%. This revealed not only the urgency of developing public demand to encourage people to get vaccinated but also the uneven distribution of the public good. Municipalities with lower vaccination coverage were anticipated to experience increased costs in public finances due to higher rates of COVID-19 infection and deaths, stemming from a smaller vaccinated population. Table 7.5 illustrates the vaccine distribution conducted by the mayors of Mexico City (CDMX). The breakdown includes the adult population aged 60 and over, the coverage percentage for the first and second doses, and the overall number of vaccines, all categorised by the mayor's office.

In practice, the Federal Vaccination Program against COVID-19 was implemented unequally between and within the different states. Data in Figures 7.4 and 7.5 come from the states in August 2021. This demonstrates the unbalanced federalism that has affected the quality and number of public policies (here measured in vaccines) available to be administered by state and municipal governments. The consequences of this imbalance were acutely evident during the COVID-19 pandemic, particularly since the largest number of patients and deaths were concentrated in Mexico City, Chihuahua, Baja California, and Sonora, which presented many more cases than in the rest of the country combined. In fact, if these states are omitted, the cases seem to be more evenly distributed with respect to the others. Also, the states with the highest accumulated case and death rates from COVID-19 are generally considered some of Mexico's wealthiest states. Few of them were part of the Federalist Alliance, which complained at the beginning of the pandemic of the lack of public policies at the national level.

Table 7.5 COVID-19 vaccination data in Mexico City (April 2021)

Mayor's office	Adult population aged 60 and over	Adult population aged 60 and over vaccinated (first dose)	Percentage of coverage (first dose)	Adult population aged 60 and over vaccinated (second dose)	Percentage of coverage (second dose)	Total vaccines
Alvaro Obregón	128,076	95,910	75%			95,910
Azcapotzalco	89,517	85,310	95%	13,748	16%	99,058
Benito Juárez	99,996	70,053	70%			70,053
Coyoacán	137,310	127,116	93%			127,116
Cuajimalpa de Morelos	26,792	29,185	109%	9,039	31%	38,224
Cuauhtémoc	110,260	75,261	68%			75,261
Gustavo A. Madero	233,866	175,040	75%			175,040
Iztacalco	79,595	71,653	90%	71,459	100%	143,112
Iztapalapa	285,263	212,368	74%			212,368
Magdalena Contreras	39,385	41,785	106%	11,780	28%	54,565
Miguel Hidalgo	76,038	89,789	118%	12,161	14%	101,950
Milpa Alta	16,870	14,340	85%	5,270	37%	19,610
Tláhuac	49,816	43,096	87%	42,322	98%	85,418
Tlalpan	114,065	90,858	80%			90,858
Venustiano Carranza	91,241	72,883	80%			72,883
Xochimilco	65,169	61,361	94%	59,992	98%	121,353
Total	1,643,259	1,356,008	83%	225,771	17%	1,581,779

Source: Author's own elaboration with data from Mexico City's Government

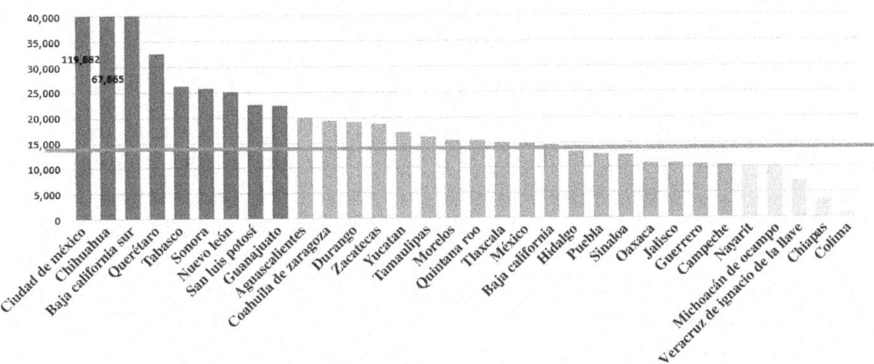

Figure 7.4 Accumulated cases of COVID-19 per million inhabitants (as of August 2021)

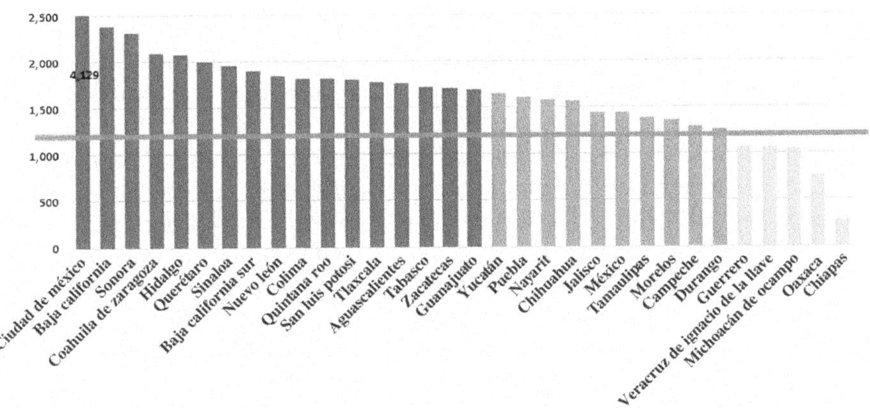

Figure 7.5 Accumulated deaths of COVID-19 per million inhabitants (as of August 2021)

Discussion and Application of Best Practices

Beginning with the official declaration of the COVID-19 pandemic by the World Health Organization (WHO) in March 2020, the Mexican presidential government's response was weak. Similar to other federalist states like the United States, Brazil, Argentina, and India, President López Obrador downplayed the pandemic, expressed scepticism, criticised mask usage, and delayed policy responses (Russell, 2020; Smith and Velázquez, 2020; Velázquez, 2020; Huerta Cuervo, 2021). In federalist countries, the pandemic highlighted the political consequences of how both the head of government and subnational governments diverged in their governing styles (Hegele and Schnabel, 2021; Ramírez de la Cruz *et al.*, 2020). This was evident in the delated governmental activities, public notifications, coercive measures for public health, and social policy responses, revealing deficiencies in the welfare state, the economy, and social policies.

In general, the global recommendation for governments was to implement a multifaceted response to the COVID-19 pandemic. Health guidelines, for example, to be issued by the Ministry of Health, emphasised practices such as social distancing, hygiene, and the use of face masks to mitigate the spread of the virus. To address the economic repercussions of the pandemic, governments were recommended to introduce measures to provide financial support for businesses, particularly small and medium-sized enterprises, and offer aid to individuals affected by the economic downturn. A critical component of the recommendations was the initiation of a nationwide vaccination campaign to reduce the severity of the disease.

Despite a delayed response, the Mexican government collaborated with international organisations like the WHO and Pan-American Health Organization to address pandemic challenges to a varying extent, as reviewed in other chapters in this volume. Regular press conferences aimed to inform the public, share health information, and address concerns. Communication channels were diversified for preventive measures, but criticisms arose regarding testing adequacy, data transparency, and delays in implementing strict measures. The initial approach focused on "flattening the curve" to prevent overwhelming hospitals. States swiftly imposed economic restrictions, many with limited resources. The government, led by Hugo López Gatell, did seek to isolate COVID-19-positive individuals; it did not emphasise testing as this was too expensive for the government to manage. As a result, independent private testing sites sprang up across the country, with tents and centres next to the airports because it was mandated abroad to have a negative test in order to fly.

Because of the late and often contradictory federal governmental response, hospital capacity was exceeded in some localities, which likely contributed to the death toll. Although some states made additional funding available for their healthcare systems and/or sought to reduce out-of-pocket healthcare costs for their citizens, their intentions were limited, and many did not take these steps at all. In addition to providing care, the ability of state governments to reduce the impact of COVID-19 on their population was probably related to their inability to coordinate health, social care services, and other forms of support. Although much of the success in containing the pandemic was due to the later vaccination campaigns, the national government often conflicted in responses to opposition governors of some states (see Table 7.6).

The crisis' enormity reveals shortcomings in Mexico's governmental failures, particularly in the design and implementation of public policies. However, it is crucial to note that the issue may lie not in the federal system's

Table 7.6 Policy outcomes

Issues	*Examples*
Hospital capacity challenges	Due to delayed federal response, some localities faced overcrowded hospitals, shortages of resources, and increased pressure on healthcare workers.
Varied state responses	While some states proactively addressed healthcare challenges, others did not allocate additional funding or prioritise reducing out-of-pocket healthcare costs.
Limited intentions and actions	Some states had limited intentions to address healthcare challenges, and certain regions took no steps at all, potentially leading to disparities in healthcare services.
Contributions to death toll	The late and contradictory federal response, coupled with varied state actions, likely contributed to higher mortality rates, especially in regions with strained healthcare systems.

Source: Own elaboration

design itself but rather in how politicians utilise available mechanisms for state coordination. In the realm of the health crisis, such mechanisms as the Consejo Nacional de Salud (CNS), which comprises all 32 heads of health services, have historically been effective in addressing health emergencies. For example, during the 2009 AH1N1 influenza outbreak, the CNS was rather successful at minimising deaths and lasted only a few weeks. Yet, interestingly, during the COVID-19 pandemic, this council appeared to be marginalised, with the president opting to delegate and centralise power in the hands of Hugo López-Gatell, Undersecretary of Health. This shift raised questions about the use of established coordination mechanisms and their effectiveness in managing crises. Therefore, this also explains not only why the governors of the Federalist Alliance took their own path, leaving the CSG and creating their own public policies, but also why they were unsuccessful in mitigating the pandemic effects and winning at the ballot box in July 2021 (see Table 7.7).

So therefore, the lack of an immediate response by the national government's social policy to attack the COVID-19 pandemic also had a direct impact on the quality of life of the population, with important distributional consequences, imposing great costs on society with little change to fiscal policy (Cardenas *et al.*, 2021). Unlike other countries, Mexico did not drastically change its fiscal accounts; instead, the government reallocated resources not used in the 2020 fiscal year and allocated them to other vital priorities such as hospitals, social policies, and other related expenses to the pandemic. The president also maintained his projects that were established at the beginning of his term: the Tren Maya in the Yucatan Peninsula, the refinery in his home state of Tabasco, and the new airport construction north of Mexico City. Huerta Cuervo (2021) revealed that the Mexican government allocated only

Table 7.7 Collaborative government failures

Issues	Examples
Delegation of power to Consejo de Salubridad general	Issue: During the pandemic, President López Obrador delegated significant power to the Consejo de Salubridad General, concentrating decision-making authority.
	Impact: Concerns about excluding the Consejo Nacional de Salud, a broader council, raised questions about inclusivity and effectiveness.
Coordination mechanisms neglect	Issue: Despite existing mechanisms like the Consejo Nacional de Salud, their effectiveness seemed compromised during the crisis.
	Impact: Neglecting established coordination mechanisms could hinder an efficient response, influencing the overall effectiveness of crisis management.
Federal-state coordination challenges	Issue: Challenges in how politicians utilise mechanisms for coordinating with states, implying coordination issues between federal and state levels.
	Impact: Inconsistencies in coordination may result in delays, gaps, or inefficiencies in crisis management, emphasising the need for smooth collaboration between government levels.
Deficiencies in the institutional federalist system	Issue: Identified deficiencies in Mexico's incomplete institutional federalist system, suggesting inherent problems.
	Impact: If the institutional design lacks the necessary elements for effective crisis management, it can impede a coordinated response, highlighting the importance of identifying and addressing these deficiencies.
Late and contradictory federal response	Issue: Hospital capacity exceeded in some localities due to late and contradictory federal response.
	Examples: Some states made additional funding available and sought to reduce out-of-pocket healthcare costs, while others had limited intentions or took no steps at all.

Source: Own elaboration

0.4% of the GDP for pandemic mitigation. She (Huerta Cuervo, 2021, p. 48) suggested that this "indicated a lack of understanding of the crisis's magnitude and its destructive impact on the economy.[5] In Mexico, 56% work in the informal sector, and 88% of companies have one to five employees, making it unrealistic to expect these businesses to maintain salaries without income." This created high levels of inequality among workers. For example, individuals or businesses whose immediate economic needs were met were more likely to be able to comply with work-from-home orders; the retaining workers had to fend for themselves in the streets.

Mexico's COVID-19 response revealed disparities in state-level actions and underscored the challenges of coordinating efforts across government levels. While subnational actors played a crucial role in implementing social policies, responses varied in type and rigour, as documented by Giraudy, Niedzwiecki and Pribble (2020) and Ramírez de la Cruz *et al.* (2020). Essential policies, such as isolation measures and vaccine coordination, were implemented by mayors and neighbourhood representatives, highlighting the importance and need for strong institutional capacity at the local level but were not sufficient for cross-state collaboration.

The fragmented subnational responses emphasise the need for a unified approach by the central government. The Federalist Alliance's actions reflected a collective action problem, revealing challenges in coordinating pandemic responses across diverse political landscapes when local control was insufficient. Examining the federalist system, this study suggests theoretical benefits of decentralisation, but practical implementation in Mexico showed imbalances with income centralisation and vaccine distribution in wealthy areas first receiving aid and treatments. This imbalance contributed to the disproportionate concentration of COVID-19 cases and deaths in specific regions, emphasising the need for a new system ensuring more equitable policy implementation.

In summary, the analysis by Hegele and Schnabel (2021) did not consider the high levels of inequality within some states, between some states, and among the greater population in such places as Mexico. Mexico therefore needed strong central government control despite government failures at all levels. The success of presidentialism, especially in times of crisis, aligns with similar research (Soto Flores, 2012; Legler, 2021), and was thus evident in the voters' decision in the July 2021 midterm election.

Conclusion

This comprehensive study delved into the complex dynamics of federalism, pandemic politics, and governance in Mexico during the COVID-19 crisis. It highlighted the Federalist Alliance's political actions, struggles over the National Conference of Governors, and electoral outcomes, collectively shaping a narrative of power dynamics amid a significant health crisis. Despite these political actions, the study emphasises the urgent need to re-evaluate and restructure the federalist system, aiming to enhance institutional capacity for future crises, delegate fiscal autonomy in policymaking, and address issues in long-term economic development and democracy under weak national governance.

The envisioned federalist system in Mexico, designed for efficiency and citizen welfare, faces practical challenges. Despite intended decentralisation, persistent fiscal imbalances have led to excessive state dependency on federal resources. The COVID-19 pandemic exacerbated these disparities, disproportionately affecting specific highly wealthy and populated states. While the decentralisation process initiated in 1989 paradoxically heightened fiscal reliance on the federal government, many poor states need federal guidance to provide effective policy implementation at the local level. States' responses during the pandemic varied substantially without clear cooperation mechanisms, revealing discrepancies in crisis-handling capacities and highlighting the need for nuanced regional strategies in social programmes.

The study underscored diverse subnational responses to COVID-19 in Mexico, exposing the absence of a unified national strategy, a lack of collaborative governance, and infighting between governors and mayors on who and how to respond to the crisis. The chapter explored relevant literature on presidentialism, governance, and federalism's limitations amid fiscal inequality. The case study on vaccine distribution in Mexico City highlights disparities, emphasising the importance of local public policy initiatives to address inequities and promote vaccination. Overall, the pandemic exposed weaknesses in Mexico's healthcare system, leading to the formation of the Federalist Alliance, which criticised federal management and advocated for regional coordination. This power struggle influenced the 2021 midterm elections, resulting in weakened decentralisation and strengthened federal control.

The study also revealed serious limitations in the presidential system in Mexico's nascent democracy. Despite democratic reforms and decentralisation, the absence of a uniform national policy response to the COVID-19 pandemic indicated major government failure to adequately address citizens' needs. This was especially the case because additional financial resources were not sought after by national authorities from the global community and were not included in the pandemic relief efforts at a national level. This resulted in a heterogeneous subnational response, as seen in the case study of vaccine distribution in Mexico City and federal social policies implemented, providing evidence of this imbalance in local-level capacities, both vertically and horizontally.

Notes

1 The first case of COVID-19 in Mexico was reported on February 21, 2020. By the end of the year, the total confirmed infections had surpassed 1.4 million, and the associated deaths were nearing 126,000. According to Statista, as of November 9, 2023, the recorded cases had surged to almost 7.7 million, with around 335,000 deaths.

2 According to Huerta Cuervo (2021, p. 48), on March 14, the first call for "*sana distancia*," or social distancing, was initiated, leading to the suspension of classes by the Ministry of Public Education from March 20 to April 20. Various organisations, including the Supreme Court of Justice of the Nation and the National Electoral Institute, shifted to virtual activities, and several large-scale events were cancelled. On March 19, following the WHO's pandemic declaration, the president mentioned preparing the DN-III Plan, involving the Army and Navy for medical support. Notably, the health sector and previous pandemic response plans were not explicitly mentioned. The government's approach lacked coordination and a unified plan among public agencies. While the effects of COVID-19 were clear in China, Europe, and New York, in Mexico they were minimised by the national response. Contradictory messages from the authorities to the population were given daily, but gradually the presidential perspective prevailed (Associated Press, 2021).

3 In his article, Frenk (2020) suggests "Another serious limitation of Insabi is that it does not have projections of what it will cost to operate it. This is a crucial variable because health officials of the current administration assure that this institute will eventually provide the same health benefits that social security institutions offer today, in particular the Mexican Social Security Institute (IMSS). However, a study carried out by analysts from the Mexican Health Foundation indicates that offering a package of health services like that of the IMSS to the 71.6 million Mexicans who do not have social security would require all the resources that were assigned to Seguro Popular (80 billion pesos) plus an additional 346 billion pesos, which represent 1.5% of GDP."

4 The Cyr *et al.* (2021) study employed newspaper clippings to assess five dimensions of collaborative governance, focusing on two key variables: inter-governmental collaboration, which evaluated policy planning and implementation involving meetings between national and subnational governments, and institutional collaboration, which examined collaboration among national ministries and/or across national and subnational bureaucracies. These include the bureaucracies (here the national ministry of health), which involve technocrats and bureaucrats with specialised knowledge in policy areas, addressing both technical and political challenges in public policymaking.

5 Huerta Cuervo (2021) cited the World Bank study *How Are We Doing* (2022), which compared Mexico to other fiscal responses like Chile (5.5%), Canada (8.4%), the United States (12.4%), Germany (32%), and Italy (12.5%), which allocated considerable resources to confront the crisis in 2020.

References

Associated Press (2021, 26 March) *México se queja de que turistas no usan mascarillas*. Available at: https://apnews.com/article/noticias-de66bac813cf417db81ec4a 762304ded (Accessed 4 August 2021).

Bodea, C. and Hicks, R. (2015) 'International finance and central bank independence: institutional diffusion and the flow and cost of capital', *Journal of Politics*, 77 pp. 268–284.

Cardenas, M. *et al.* (2021) 'Fiscal policy challenges for Latin America during the next stages of the pandemic: the need for a Fiscal pact', *IMF Working Papers*, 2021(77), p. A001. Available at: www.elibrary.imf.org/view/journals/001/2021/077/article-A001-en.xml (Accessed 3 August 2021).

Consejo Nacional de Ciencia y Tecnología (2020) *Mapa y casos de coronavirus en México por estados*. Available at: https://datos.covid-19.conacyt.mx/ (Acceso 29 octubre 2020).

Consejo Nacional de Ciencia y Tecnología (Conacyt) (2021) 'Información general COVID-19 México,' *Electrónico*. Available at: https://datos.covid-19.conacyt.mx/ (Accessed 8 June 2021).

Consejo Nacional de Evaluación de la Política del Desarrollo Social (2020) *La crisis sanitaria generada por la COVID-19*. Available at: www.coneval.org.mx/Evaluacion/IEPSM/Paginas/Politica_Social_COVID-19.aspx (Acceso 29 octubre 2020).

Cyr, J. *et al.* (2021) 'Governing a pandemic: assessing the role of collaboration on Latin American responses to the COVID-19 crisis', *Journal of Politics in Latin America*, 13(3), pp. 290–327. https://doi.org/10.1177/1866802X211049250.

Diaz-Cayeros, A. (2006) *Federalism, fiscal authority, and centralization in Latin America*. Cambridge, New York: Cambridge University Press. Available at: https://datos.bancomundial.org/indicator/NY.GDP.MKTP.CD.

Frenk, J. and Gómez Dantés, O. (2020, 26 May) *Salud: La democratización interrumpida*. Mexico City: Letras Libres. Available at: https://letraslibres.com/politica/salud-la-democratizacion-interrumpida/ (Accessed 14 December 2023).

Gandarilla, N. (2012) *Efecto flypaper en el gasto público de los Estados en México*. Mexico City: ITESM-EGAP. Available at: https://repositorio.tec.mx/bitstream/handle/11285/629331/33068001103103.pdf?sequence=1&isAllowed=y.

Giraudy, A., Niedzwiecki, S. and Pribble, J. (2020, 30 April) 'How political science explains countries' reactions to COVID-19', *Americas Quarterly*. Available at: www.americasquarterly.org/article/how-political-science-explains-countries-reactions-to-covid-19/.

Hegele, Y. and Schnabel, J. (2021) 'Federalism and the management of the COVID-19 crisis: centralisation, decentralisation, and (non-)coordination', *West European Politics*, 44(5–6), pp. 1052–1076. https://doi.org/10.1080/01402382.2021.1873529.

Hernández-Trillo, F. (2018) 'When lack of accountability allows observing unobservables: moral hazard in sub-national government credit markets in Mexico', *Applied Economics Letters*, 25(5), pp. 326–330. https://doi.org/10.1080/13504851.2017.1321828.

Hopkins, J. (2020, 23 octubre) *Coronavirus resource center*. de John Hopkins University and Medicine. Disponible en: https://coronavirus.jhu.edu/map.html.

Huerta Cuervo, Rocío (2021) 'Vicisitudes en la Gestión de la pandemia por COVID19 en México', in Espinosa Castillo, M., Rivera, A. and Aguilar, M. (eds.) *Implicaciones y oportunidades de la emergencia sanitaria por COVID19*. Madrid: Editorial Diaz de Santos, pp. 41–56.

Jimenez Quiroga, C.I. and Smith, H.J.M. (2019) 'Incentivos buenos e incentivos perversos en México', *Un Análisis del patrón de endeudamiento subnacional Pluralidad y Consenso*, 9(40), pp. 104–112. ISSN: 2395-8138.

Knaul, F.M. *et al.* (2023) 'Setbacks in the quest for universal health coverage in Mexico: polarised politics, policy upheaval, and pandemic disruption', *Lancet. Health Policy*, 402(10403), pp. 731–746. https://doi.org/10.1016/S0140-6736(23)00777-8.

LaboratorioNacional de Políticas Públicas de CIDE (2020) *Medidas económicas ante la pandemia por COVID-19*. Available at: https://mexico.as.com/mexico/2020/10/20/actualidad/1603200397_158976.html (Acceso 29 octubre 2020).

LaboratorioNacional de Políticas Públicas de CIDE (2021) *Mapa de medidas económicas ante a pandemia por COVID-19, ¿Qué hacen los estados frente a la crisis económica provocada por COVID-19?* Available at: https://lnpp.cide.edu/proyectos/4 (Accessed 8 June 2021).

Legler, T. (2021, abril—junio). 'Presidentes y orquestadores: la gobernanza de la pandemia de Covid-19 en las Américas', *Foro Internacional*, LXI(2), p. 244. https://doi.org/10.24201/fi.v61i2.2833.

Lehoucq, F. *et al.* (2005) 'Policymaking in Mexico under one-party hegemony and divided government', in Stein, E., Tommasi, M., Scartascini, C. and Spiller, P. (eds.) *Policymaking in Latin America: how politics shapes policies*. Washington, DC: Banco Interamericano de Desarrollo. Available at: www.iadb.org/res/pub_desc.cfm?pub_id=R-512.

Medrano, A. (2016) 'Social policy innovation at state-level: an analytical framework for the case of Mexico', *Journal of Public Governance and Policy: Latin American Review*, 1(4), pp. 51–72.

Medrano, A. and Smith, H.J.M. (2017) 'State investment in social programs after three decades of decentralization and social reform in Mexico', *Gestión y Políticas Pública*, 26, pp. 157–189. [Online]. ISSN: 1405-1079.

Mendoza-Velázquez, A. (2018) *Los incentivos perversos del Federalismo fiscal mexicano México*. Mexico City: Colección Lecturas del Trimestre Económico (FCE). Available at: www.fondodeculturaeconomica.com/Ficha/9786071661807/F.

Moreno Jaimes, C., Rojas-Alvarez, A. and Angel, J.L. (2023, 23 August) *Del Seguro Popular al Insabi: efectos de la recentralización parcial sobre la cobertura de servicios de salud*. Mexico City: Nexus. Available at: https://federalismo.nexos.com.

mx/2023/08/del-seguro-popular-al-insabi-efectos-de-la-recentralizacion-parcial-sobre-la-cobertura-de-servicios-de-salud/ (Accessed 14 December 2023).

Mosley, L. (2000) 'Room to move: international financial markets and national welfare states', *International Organization,* 54, pp. 737–774.

Oates, W.E. (1972) *Fiscal federalism.* New York: Harcourt Brace Jovanovich.

Observatorio Covid-19 (2021) *Índice de adopción de políticas públicas.* Available at: http://observcovid.miami.edu/mexico/?lang=es.

Our World in Data (2021) 'Covid-19 cases', *Electrónico.* Disponible en: https://our worldindata.org/covid-cases (Acceso 8 junio 2021).

Pérez Benítez, N. and Villarreal Páez, H.J. (2018) 'El espacio fiscal de los estados. Definiciones e implicaciones', in Mendoza Velázquez, A. (ed.) *Los incentivos perversos del Federalismo fiscal mexicano. La necesidad de un nuevo modelo.* Ciudad de México: Fondo de Cultura Económica.

Periódico el Heraldo (2021) 'Pandemia de Covid-19 evidencia la inequidad del Federalismo en México: Expertos', *Heraldo de Mexico.* Available at: https://her aldodemexico.com.mx/nacional/2021/3/18/pandemia-de-covid-19-evidencia-la-inequidad-del-Federalismo-en-mexico-expertos-272298.html.

Pliego Moreno, I. (2012) 'El Federalismo fiscal en México: entre la economía y la política', in Meixueiro Nájera, G. (ed.) *Desarrollo regional y agenda legislativa,* Mexico City: Centro de Estudios Sociales y de Opinión Pública/Cámara de Diputados, LXI Legislatura, pp. 195–228.

Portal Ciudadano Gobierno Ciudad de México (2021) Available at: https://datos. covid-19.conacyt.mx/ www.cdmx.gob.mx/ (Accessed 18 June 2021).

Ramírez de la Cruz, E.E. *et al.* (2020) 'The transaction costs of government responses to the COVID-19 emergency in Latin America', *Public Administration Review,* 80, pp. 683–695. https://doi.org/10.1111/puar.13259.

Rodríguez, R. (1998) 'El Presidencialismo Mexicano, ¿Cuánto Es Indispensable Limitarlo?', in Migallón, F. (ed.) *Homenaje a Rafael Segovia.* México, DF: El Colegio de Mexico, pp. 193–210. https://doi.org/10.2307/j.ctv3f8pnn.12.

Rogers, M.Z. *et al.* (2021) 'Inequality in risk-taking: evidence from location tracking in Mexican cities during COVID-19', *Frontiers in Political Science,* 3, p. 631826. https://doi.org/10.3389/fpos.2021.631826.

Rosenbaum, A. and Rodriguez Acosta, C. (2008) 'Metropolitan governments in Latin America', in De Vries, M., Reddy, P. and Samsul Haque, M. (eds.) *Improving local government: outcomes of comparative research.* New York, NY: Palgrave Macmillan.

Russell, B. (2020, 21 April) *Mexico's governors find their voice—and the spotlight—in COVID-19.* Available at: www.americasquarterly.org/article/mexicos-governors-find-their-voice-and-the-spotlight-in-covid-19/.

Smith, H.J.M. (2018) 'Aumento de la capacidad de toma de decisiones de los gobiernos locales: la búsqueda de crecimiento económico de México', in Mendoza Velázquez, A. (coord.) *Los incentivos perversos del Federalismo fiscal mexicano, Trimestre Económico.* Mexico City: FCE, pp. 127–162. ISBN: 978-607-16-6039-7.

Smith, H.J.M. and Revell, K. (2016) 'Micro-incentives and municipal behavior: political decentralization and Fiscal federalism in Argentina and Mexico', *World Development,* 77, pp. 231–248.

Smith, H.J.M. and Velázquez, C. (2020, 7 May) 'La pandemia y el Federalismo en México', *Sobre Mexico Blog.* Universidad Iberoamericana. Available at: https:// blog.economia.ibero.mx/la-pandemia-y-el-Federalismo-en-mexico\.

Soto Flores, A. (2012) 'El presidencialismo mexicano en los umbrales del siglo XXI. del sistema presidencialista hacia un sistema presidencial con matices parlamentarios', *Revista de la Facultad de Derecho de México,* 61(256), pp. 305–320. https://doi.org/10.22201/fder.24488933e.2011.256.30377.

Sour, L. (2008) *El enfoque económico en el estudio de las políticas públicas*. CIDE, p. 206. Disponible en: http://libreriacide.com/librospdf/DTAP-206.pdf.

Tan, E. and Avshalom-Uster, A. (2021) 'How does asymmetric decentralization affect local fiscal performance?', *Regional Studies*, 55(6), pp. 1071–1083. https://doi.org/10.1080/00343404.2020.1861241.

Tanzi, V. (2000) '*On Fiscal federalism: issues to worry about*'. Available at: https://www.imf.org/external/pubs/ft/seminar/2000/fiscal/tanzi.pdf.

Velázquez, C. (2020, 21 August) 'El pacto fiscal y las participaciones Federales', *Sobre Mexico Blog*. Universidad Iberoamericana. Available at: https://blog.economia.ibero.mx/el-pacto-fiscal-y-las-participaciones-Federales/.

Weldon, J. (1997) 'Political sources of Presidencialismo in Mexico', in Mainwaring, S. and Shugart, M. (eds.) *Presidentialism and democracy in Latin America (Cambridge studies in comparative politics)*. Cambridge: Cambridge University Press, pp. 225–258. https://doi.org/10.1017/CBO9781139174800.007.

Wiesner, E. (2003) *Fiscal federalism in Latin America from entitlements to markets*. Washington, DC: Inter-American Development Bank Distributed by the Johns Hopkins University Press.

8 Conclusion, It's the Politics, Stupid

The Challenge of Minimising
Their Negative Impact on Future
Pandemics

Thomas Legler

It's the politics, stupid! The authors in this volume have highlighted in diverse ways how deleterious forms of pandemic politics contributed to Mexico's painful experience with COVID-19. Mexicans paid a heavy price in terms of unnecessary human suffering because both global governance and governmental authorities on many accounts got the politics of the pandemic response wrong. Importantly, it was not necessarily global and domestic policies in themselves that were at fault, but how they were politicised. Counterfactually, in a country that ranked fifth in the world for the most COVID-19 deaths, many Mexican lives could have been saved if the Mexican government and global governance actors had gotten the politics right (Dávila, 2023; Latinus, 2023; Sánchez Talanquer and Sepúlveda, 2024).

What do we mean when we say that these actors got the politics wrong? Throughout the pages of this book, the authors have offered a select set of vignettes that illustrate how different forms of politics got in the way of protecting the health and lives of Mexicans. In our texts, we assign blame to the politics of both global governance and domestic governmental processes during the COVID-19 crisis and the interactions between the two.

For example, Laura Zamudio observes how the symbolic politics perpetrated by the Mexican government sewed discord with and hurt the attempts by the World Health Organization (WHO) to fill the enormous knowledge gap regarding COVID-19 that existed with consensual and reliable meanings and understandings based on scientific evidence. In their chapter, Valeria Valle, Caroline Deschak, and Michelle Ruiz tell of how informal and formal types of disease diplomacy, as well as discriminatory intersectional politics, affected the access of migrants to COVID-19-related health services along the border in the vicinity of Tijuana during the pandemic.

Various contributors, including Laura Zamudio, Maria Esther Coronado, Thomas Legler, Gabriela Palacios, and Ricardo Velázquez, underline the damaging effects of medical populism as it was practiced in Mexico. In addition to promoting discretionary decision-making and de-institutionalisation, populist impulses underpinned the centralisation and politicisation of public health measures, which came at the expense of more comprehensive, coordinated, and integrated whole-of-government and whole-of-society approaches

DOI: 10.4324/9781003494959-8

to the pandemic. In this regard, Heidi Smith's chapter recounts how Mexico's federal system, which in theory should have performed much better, in practice became the terrain for federal-state political conflict. According to Laura Zamudio, populist governments also severely limited the efficacy of governance orchestration by the WHO.

The contributions also find fault with the global governance side of the equation. For instance, Maria Esther Coronado exposes the politicisation and resulting division of the epistemic communities upon which the WHO relied for the development and dissemination of its global health policies and recommendations, thanks to the juxtaposition of transnational expert and transgovernmental networks and the dual role of scientists as specialists and bureaucrats. In terms of the global political economy of pandemic responses, Legler's chapter emphasises how asymmetries of political and economic power helped fashion a global vaccine governance complex that accentuated rather than reduced global vaccine inequity. This put the onus on countries like Mexico to adopt the pragmatic measures necessary in order to obtain an adequate and reliable vaccine supply. In their comparison of governmental responses to the pandemic in Ecuador and Mexico, Palacios and Velázquez share how the actions of some international organisations, namely, the International Monetary Fund, may act against the building up of resilient health systems against public health emergencies. They also highlight the frequent contradictions and lack of coordination in the global policies of these organisations.

Have global governors and governments learnt the political lessons of the pandemic? If the current negotiation process for a new pandemic treaty is any indication, the answer is no. In December 2021, a special World Health Assembly (WHA) formally created an Intergovernmental Negotiating Body (INB) to craft an international agreement whose purpose was to strengthen the global governance of pandemic preparedness, detection, and response in light of the world's recent experience with COVID-19. After more than two years of continuous talks, the INB failed to meet its May 24, 2024 deadline for producing an agreement, prompting the members of the WHA to establish a new target date of June 2025. As one source remarked, "the world seems to be seeking to fix political problems with technical solutions. The problems which determined the failures of global action during Covid were wholly political." These same authors criticised that precisely what was missing from the discussions was attention to the political and that what is required are political and not technical solutions (Wenham and Eccleston-Turner, 2024, p. 1).

One of the clear deficiencies of the treaty negotiation process is the lack of determination to address sovereignty politics, or what some scholars have termed the statist versus globalist tension (Wenham, Eccleston-Turner and Voss, 2022). Concretely, the reluctance of member states to cede their sovereign authority over health security in relation to threats from viruses with pandemic potential severely weakened attempts within the INB to create a robust treaty compliance mechanism, the Implementation and Compliance Committee. A proposal for an independent global system of monitoring and peer review was cut in favour of a watered-down mechanism whose efforts would focus on the "facilitation" and "promotion" of "non-adversarial" compliance measures (Schwalbe, Hannon and Lehtimaki, 2024).

Despite plenty of rhetoric in favour of greater equity in the global governance of pandemics, the negotiations have also failed to attack the global political economy roots of inequity in global and national responses to contagious diseases. Thus far, the talks have failed to make significant advances in terms of more equitable access to countermeasures, such as medicines and vaccines. There is little agreement on the question of the redistribution of medical supplies and vaccines, as well as technology transfer, enhancing manufacturing capacity, and financing for middle- and low-income countries (Taylor, 2024; Wenham and Eccleston-Turner, 2024).

Accordingly, the status quo that prevailed during COVID-19 appears alive and well. That is, states persist in their reluctance to delegate sovereign authority in questions of health security and a privileged set of countries and economic interests located predominantly in the Global North continue to enjoy and concentrate disproportionate influence and benefits from the existing global health governance architecture, to the detriment of the poorer countries and populations of the Global South.

But what does it mean to get the politics right? Although we do not necessarily provide definitive answers, the analyses in this volume based on the Mexican experience suggest at least three core challenges in order to point pandemic politics in the right direction. The first question is how to shield or insulate key global governance and government actors and institutions from populist politics. Insights from Mexico reveal that on the one hand, the WHO was hamstrung in its efforts to provide continuous guidance during the pandemic thanks to the challenges and select compliance that came from governments like that of López Obrador. On the other hand, the Mexican government emasculated the very governmental institutions that had been expressly created to manage public health emergencies, the General Health Council and the National Health Council.

A second challenge relates to global political economy: how to promote more equitable global pandemic governance. As mentioned earlier, there is rhetorical recognition in the current pandemic negotiation process of the need for greater equity and access for poorer countries and peoples to crucial inputs for health security in the face of pandemic threats, including medicines, medical equipment and materials, vaccines, technology, and manufacturing capacity. Sadly, the success of an eventual pandemic accord in this regard will depend to some extent on a leap of faith: that the very countries and companies that have most dominated and benefitted until now from the unequal and unjust status quo are the ones that are called upon to transform global health governance and redistribute its benefits and protections more equitably and fairly.

Lastly, in light of the multiple problems identified in this book in terms of the record of Mexican public authorities with respect to pandemic management, there is the question of how to promote greater governmental accountability and transparency, both during pandemic emergencies and in their aftermath. Thus far, the present constellation of political forces in the Mexican Chamber of Deputies and the Senate has meant that there has still not been any official public inquiry into Mexico's pandemic record. President López Obrador has certainly not shown any willingness to review his government's performance. Until now, there has only been one single attempt by a civil society initiative comprised of leading experts to hold authorities accountable: the Independent Commission on the COVID-19 Pandemic in Mexico (see Sánchez Talanquer and Sepúlveda, 2024). Even the launch of the report of this Commission failed to convert the June 2024 presidential elections into a referendum on the government's handling of the pandemic. Consequently, there is still very much a need for an open, transparent, and constructive national public inquiry that examines both the governance and governmental dimensions of the collective responses to the pandemic. It is our hope that this book makes a modest contribution toward inducing global and Mexican authorities, whether openly or discretely, to reflect on the political lessons of their management during COVID-19 before the next great one arrives.

References

Dávila, P. (2023) 'COVID-19: los pecados de López-Gatell que la Fiscalía debe investigar', *Proceso*, 10 June. Available at: www.proceso.com.mx/reportajes/2023/6/10/covid-19-los-pecados-de-lopez-gatell-que-la-fiscalia-debe-investigar-308589.html.

Latinus (2023) 'Con autorización de uso del remdesivir, el gobierno de AMLO hubiera evitado miles de muertes por Covid, acusa el doctor Francisco Moreno', *Latinus*, 13 March. Available at: https://latinus.us/2023/03/13/gobierno-amlo-muertes-covid-autorizacion-remdesivir-doctor-francisco-moreno/.

Sánchez Talanquer, M. and Sepúlveda, J. (eds.) (2024) *Informe de la Comisión Independiente de Investigación sobre la Pandemia de Covid-19 en México*. Mexico City. Available at: www.comisioncovid.mx/.

Schwalbe, N., Hannon, E. and Lehtimaki, S. (2024, 22 February) 'The new pandemic treaty: are we in safer hands? Probably not', *British Medical Journal*, 384, p. q477. Available at: www.bmj.com/content/bmj/384/bmj.q477.full.pdf.

Taylor, L. (2024, 4 June) 'WHO member states agree better ways to detect health threats and set new deadline for pandemic treaty', *British Medical Journal*, 385, p. q1227. Available at: www.bmj.com/content/bmj/385/bmj.q1227.full.pdf.

Wenham, C. and Eccleston-Turner, M. (2024, 15 February) 'Will the pandemic treaty make it over the line?', *British Medical Journal*, 384, p. q395. Available at: www.bmj.com/content/bmj/384/bmj.q395.full.pdf.

Wenham, C., Eccleston-Turner, M. and Voss, M. (2022) 'The futility of the pandemic treaty: caught between globalism and statism', *International Affairs*, 98(3), pp. 837–852.

Index

Note: Page numbers in *italic* indicate a figure and page numbers in **bold** indicate a table on the corresponding page.

For Product Safety Concerns and Information please contact our EU
representative GPSR@taylorandfrancis.com
Taylor & Francis Verlag GmbH, Kaufingerstraße 24, 80331 München, Germany

www.ingramcontent.com/pod-product-compliance
Ingram Content Group UK Ltd.
Pitfield, Milton Keynes, MK11 3LW, UK
UKHW022337100726
473146UK00010B/824